total
massage

total
massage

gill tree

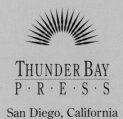

THUNDER BAY
P·R·E·S·S

San Diego, California

Caution:
This book is intended as an informational guide only and is not to be used as a substitute for professional medical care or treatment. Neither the author nor the publishers can be held responsible for any damage, injury, or otherwise resulting from the use of the information in this book.

Dedication
Total Massage is dedicated to the tutors and staff who work at my company, Essentials for Health. Their energy and inspiration has ensured that the healing power of touch is being spread throughout the world. By teaching people to be therapists and teachers, the influence of Essentials for Health works like ripples on a pond, forever emanating outward in ever-increasing circles, influencing the health and relationships of thousands of people. Thank you.

With thanks to Alan Rowe; Marie Ortu; Amanda Bradley; Aimée Burry; Caron Ladkin and Daniel Schoneveld; Tessa Landers; Heidi, Devon and Millar Vitalis; and Michelle and Amelia Dobney.

Thunder Bay Press
An imprint of the Advantage Publishers Group
THUNDER BAY   5880 Oberlin Drive, San Diego, CA 92121-4794
P·R·E·S·S   www.thunderbaybooks.com

SERIES EDITOR **Karen Ball, MQ Publications**
EDITORIAL DIRECTOR **Ljiljana Baird, MQ Publications**
PHOTOGRAPHY **Johnny Ring**
DESIGN CONCEPT **Balley Design Associates**
DESIGN **Jo Hill**
ILLUSTRATION **Oxford Designers and Illustrators**

All notations of errors or omissions should be addressed to Thunder Bay Press, Editorial Department, at the above address. All other correspondence (author inquiries, permissions) concerning the content of this book should be addressed to MQ Publications, 12 The Ivories, 6-8 Northampton Street, London N1 2HY, England.

Library of Congress Cataloging-in-Publication Data

Tree, Gill.
   Total massage / Gill Tree.
      p. cm.
   ISBN 1-59223-294-9
      1. Massage. I. Title.

RA780.5.T74 2004
613.7'2--dc22

2004047970

Printed in China
1 2 3 4 5 08 07 06 05 04

contents

introduction to massage

I believe we are all already experts when it comes to loving touch. Each of us is able to instinctively reach out and communicate through our hands what words cannot express: a deep level of feeling, understanding, and care to those we cherish.

We have all experienced the joy, security, and warmth of a welcoming embrace, the soothing strokes over the brow during illness, and the comfort of touch as someone consoles us in times of anguish. When we bang an elbow, we rub it to make it feel better without thinking, and we rush to soothe the grazed knee of a child.

Infants who do not receive loving touch can wither away and die. Adults who do not receive loving touch may become withdrawn and anxious. We can see extremes of this in those with mental illness who may slowly rock themselves for comfort. In my work as a massage therapist, I have worked with elderly people, massaging, soothing, and reducing pain in arthritic and stiff joints. I have taught the parents of premature babies how to touch their tiny children through the doors of

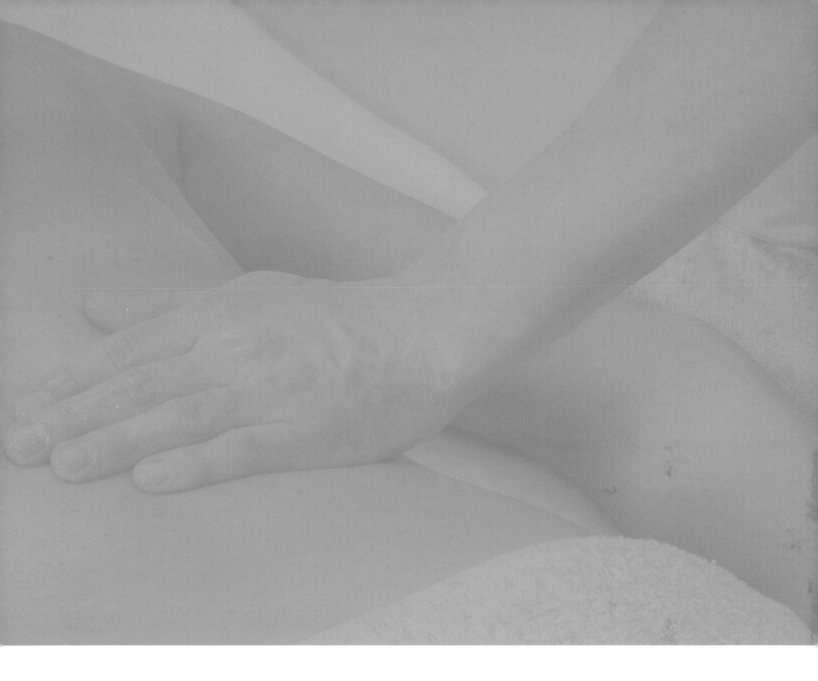

an incubator, and I have soothed dying cancer patients through their pain and suffering.

In everyday life, we can all benefit from massage therapy to help us deal with the everyday strains and stresses of modern life. Giving and receiving massage can transport both giver and recipient into an altered, meditative state. And in our fast-track, instant-gratification society, we owe it to ourselves and to our loved ones once again just to be. This book will give you some more tools to add to your instinctive touch toolbox, to enhance the quality, power, and effects of what you already do. Practice them regularly, and the techniques you learn from this book will guarantee you closer relationships with more people in your life.

When we give a massage we devote attention, time, and love to another person. Throughout our lives, in sickness and in health, the healing power of touch is there, allowing everyone to give comfort, love, support, release, and healing.

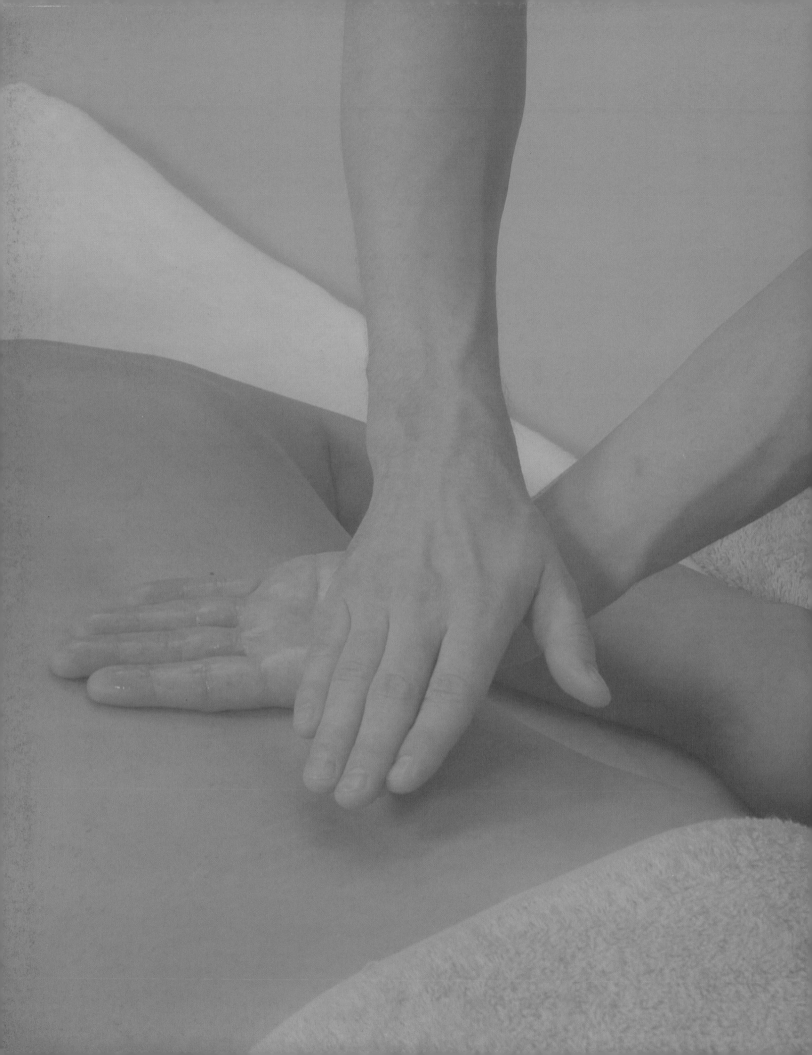

principles and background

Here you will find all the essentials you need to know before starting to give a massage: how to set up a comfortable treatment room, ways to use oil, and techniques for maintaining good posture as you work. Accompanying these basic how-tos is information on the long history and benefits of this most relaxing of complementary therapies.

how to use this book

Once you have read this first chapter, which sets out the background and philosophy of massage and offers tips on tools and preparation, you are ready to go. To make your massage life easy and rewarding, you will find in Part 2 a set menu of techniques that can be applied to any part of the body. These fundamentals can be learned within an hour or so, allowing you to quickly and effortlessly give a full-body massage without having to pore over the pages of the book, distracting from the quality of what you do.

Part 3 offers variations for each body part to add to your repertoire of strokes as and when you feel ready. Again, most of these techniques can be learned in advance through self-massage practice and by going through the motions of the techniques in the air. In Parts 4 and 5, you will find a series of distinct massage tools and techniques that encompass every stage of life from birth to the grave. These can be dipped into and enjoyed whenever appropriate in your life situation.

have fun!

I believe we should take massage seriously and treat the techniques and the person receiving them with reverence. Yet massage is also a tool to have fun with and it can generate playfulness. Once you have noted the guidance on when not to give massage on pages 38–39, the only rule of massage is to enjoy giving and receiving it. Your way of doing it is the right way, so take what fits your particular likes and dislikes and go play.

the healing power of touch

Massage	Healing and health
The merging of science and art	Intoxicating and harmonizing.
The union of mind, body, and spirit	It is touch It is communication It is love made visible It is meditation in motion.
Unifying the senses	
It is stillness and movement	
Soothing and stimulating	We dance with a partner and join them in love An energy collaboration of healing, peace, tranquility, oneness, inspiration, intuition, meditation, joy, and transformation.
Yin and yang	
Calming and invigorating	It is timeless, boundless, limitless Bonding, connecting, nurturing.
Nurturing and revitalizing	
Energizing and transforming	Heavy hands, warm hands, healing hands, loving hands Repair, renew, revitalize, rejuvenate.

Gill Tree

right: Massage is an intensely satisfying and relaxing experience, for both the massage therapist and the person receiving the massage.

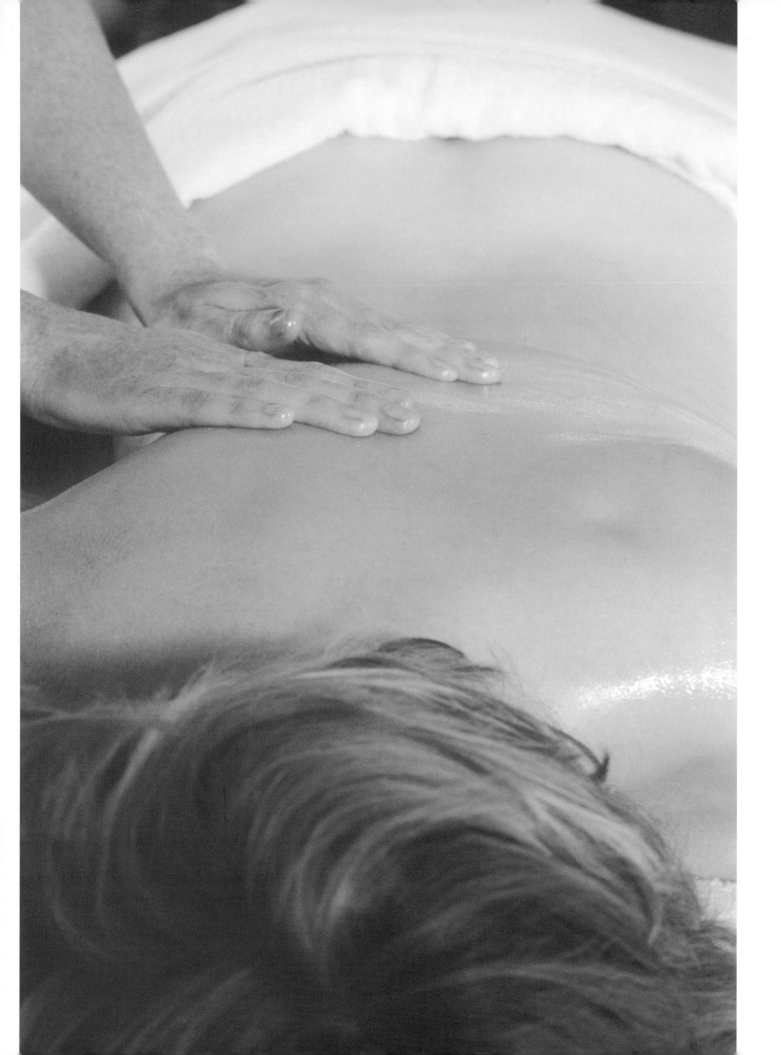

massage in the beginning

We are indebted to ancient cave dwellers and their paintings for the earliest evidence of massage in use. Wall drawings and paintings show people massaging each other. The Bible and the Qur'an refer to the use of fats and aromatic oils for anointing and lubricating the body.

The Chinese had a system of *somato,* or massage therapy, as early as 5000 BC. The oldest recorded medical text, the *Nei Jing,* dating to between c. 200 BC and AD 100, includes numerous references to the use of massage for healing purposes. Along with other forms of Traditional Chinese Medicine, the Japanese inherited massage techniques from the Chinese around 1,500 years ago. Their primary practitioners, many of them blind, had for years practiced and understood the importance of using massage in treating illness. It was further developed using similar pressure techniques on specific energy points known as *tsubos,* or acupoints. This style of massage, used through the centuries, was rediscovered in the early years of the twentieth century by practitioner Tamai Tempaku and developed into the massage form known today as shiatsu. Ancient Egyptians and Persians used massage for

below: This nineteenth-century photograph shows a Japanese shampooer massaging the back of a woman. Shampooing was an early massage technique and the precursor to some of today's modern massages. Shampooers were almost always blind, which accentuated their sense of touch.

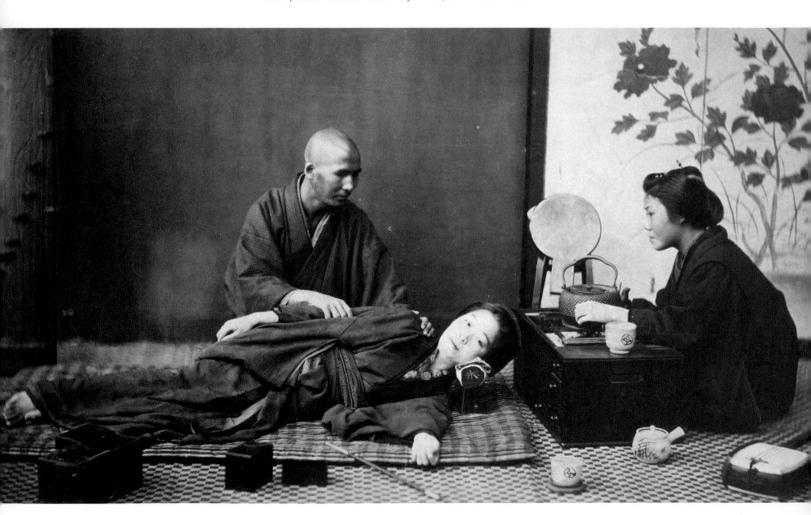

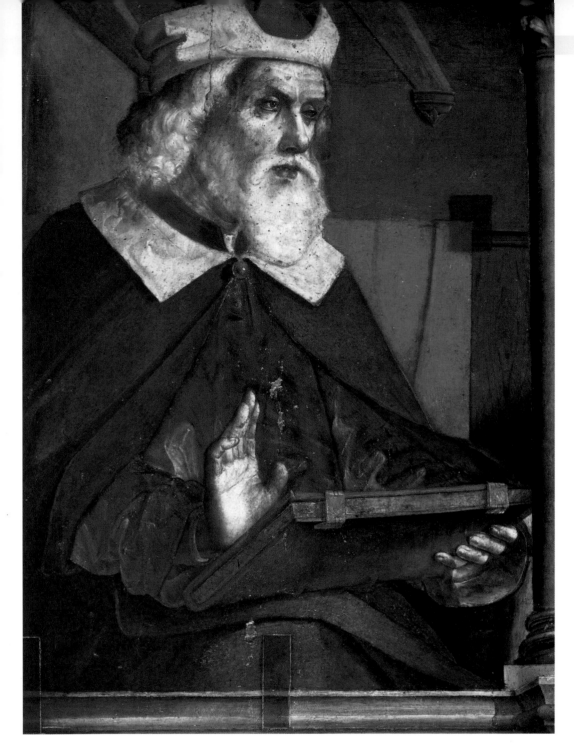

left: The Greek physician Hippocrates provided one of the first written records of the benefits of massage.

cosmetic and therapeutic effects, mixing fats, herbs, oils, and resins for skin care and beautifying the face and body. Pots and jars containing such creams were discovered in Egyptian tombs. Depictions on a wall painting of a hand and foot massage at the entrance of a physician's tomb in Saqqara date back to 2330 BC. After bathing in milk, Cleopatra was massaged by her handmaidens with aromatic oils and creams. The sacred Hindu texts, the Vedas, or books of knowledge, which began to be composed before 1200 BC, include the sacred book of ayurveda (the knowledge of living). This contains passages describing how shampooing and rubbing can reduce fatigue and promote well-being and cleanliness.

The virtues of massage were advocated by Greek thinkers such as Socrates, Plato, and Herodotus. In 5 BC, Greek physician Hippocrates (now known as the "father of medicine") was recorded as saying, "Rubbing can bind a joint that is too loose and loosen a joint that is too rigid," and "Anyone wishing to study medicine must study the art of massage." He pointed out the benefits of massage for relieving strain, constipation, and other conditions.

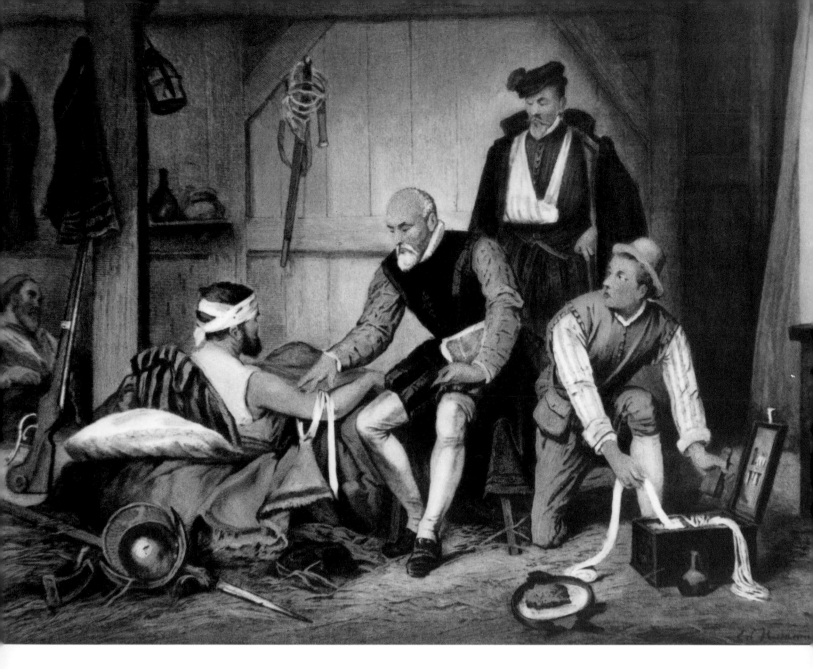

above: Abroise Paré, pictured here, was a sixteenth-century French doctor who helped develop massage into a recognized, beneficial technique for treating patients.

The Romans had a similar understanding to the Greeks, and they incorporated massage into their bathing routines. Servants would be in attendance to massage their masters and mistresses with oils and creams. Massage techniques involving manipulations such as squeezing, pummeling, and pinching directly relate to the percussion and pettrisage movements of today. To ease Julius Caesar's neuralgia and epilepsy, he was given "pinching" treatments each day. Pliny, a first-century Roman naturalist and encyclopedist, rubbed for the relief of chronic asthma, and Galen, a Roman emperor's physician in the second century, reported that gladiators were "anointed with oil and rubbed until red." He also was reputed to have said, "Massage eliminates the waste products of nutrition and the poisons of fatigue." This was incredibly accurate; massage does stimulate the digestive system, improve elimination, and encourage the removal of lactic acid, a waste product produced in muscles.

The sixteenth-century French surgeon Abroise Paré promoted and developed massage by grading strokes into gentle, medium, and vigorous. He was reported to have successfully treated Mary, Queen of Scots, with massage. Many physicians copied his methods and massage became established medically. In 1779, Captain James Cook recorded how his painful sciatica was relieved when Tahitian women gently massaged him.

Europe saw a rise in the popularity of massage during the nineteenth century when Swedish gymnast Per Henrik Ling developed a system of massage movements and coined terminology still used in massage today, including "pettrisage," "friction," and "rolling." Institutes of massage were opened in Stockholm, and in London in 1838, and Ling's students continued to make known his methods long after his death. "Swedish massage" is the term used today to describe the style of massage most commonly taught and the term used in this book. By the end of the nineteenth century, massage had become a popular medical treatment and was regularly being used by eminent surgeons, cardiologists, and physicians.

John Grosvenor, a nineteenth-century English surgeon, used massage to treat joints and recommended it to ease rheumatism, gout, and joint stiffness. Around the same time, Dutch physician Johann Mezgner combined massage techniques with his knowledge of anatomy and physiology, and his theories became accepted by the medical establishment. Massage as a therapy grew in popularity during the twentieth century, and technical progress led to the invention of mechanical massage instruments. However, proponents of traditional massage emphasize that the benefits to be gained from massage derive not only from the manipulation of muscle, but from the simplest of things—the physical touch of one human being by another.

below: The basic principle of touch between one human being and another is key to the philosophy and benefits of massage.

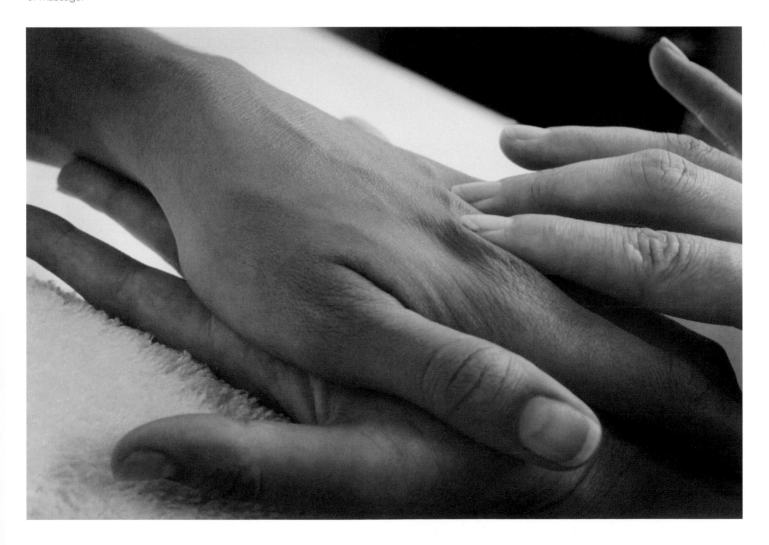

the benefits of physical touch

When one person touches another in a loving way, there is a release in both partners of the hormone oxytocin. Known to be found in abundance in breast-feeding mothers, this is the hormone that ensures that the bond with and love for the infant is secured. When released through touch in men and women, oxytocin gives us a feeling of well-being and of being nurtured. In this way, a massage treatment reaches the whole person, communicating a sense of peace and tranquility and developing inner contentment and a feeling of being in touch with our inner selves.

In all complementary therapies, there is a premise that the body is naturally designed to be in a state of ease and effortless functioning, known as homeostasis, or balance. Massage can literally soothe the nerves, produce a feeling of well-being, and bring body and mind into equilibrium. Often, after a number of massages, people find they are more aware of the body and more able to relax, switch off from intrusive thoughts, and retreat from the stress of the day. This helps to relieve mental and emotional tension that frequently manifests as tense muscles. The action of rubbing the skin also creates changes in the body that lead to the release of endorphin hormones. These are the body's natural painkillers, which also bring about the feel-good factor. All the benefits of massage help the recipient gain a realization of how good a relaxed body can feel.

physical benefits

Massage improves circulation by assisting the flow of blood from the limbs back to the heart. Deep stroking movements called "effleurage" increase the flow of fresh blood, carrying nutrients and oxygen to organs and muscles.

Massage of the abdomen stimulates the muscles of the stomach, intestines, and bowel, increasing the action of peristalsis by which food is digested. If food can be processed and eliminated more quickly, there will be fewer toxins within the body and less disease-causing bacteria.

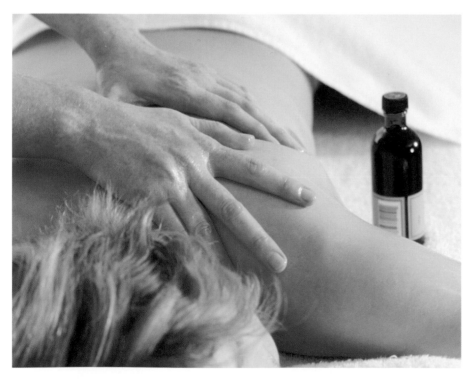

Massage encourages muscles to relax and lengthen (imagine a wound-up rubber band being unraveled), relieving tightness and tension and promoting the elimination of toxins. It also encourages fresh blood into areas of congestion, bringing fresh nutrients and oxygen to fatigued muscles and assisting with the removal of lactic acid, the toxic waste produced by muscle action. If left within a tight muscle, this waste product can crystallize and cause severe muscle soreness.

Massage assists in the flow of the straw-colored fluid known as "lymph" that circulates within the body. The lymphatic system is instrumental in fighting infection and developing immunity. Lymph nodes act as filters to prevent the spread of infection, while lymphocytes carried in the lymph fight infection. Muscular contraction, gravity, and passive movement

left: Massage allows muscles to relax, improves circulation, and aids the removal of toxic waste.

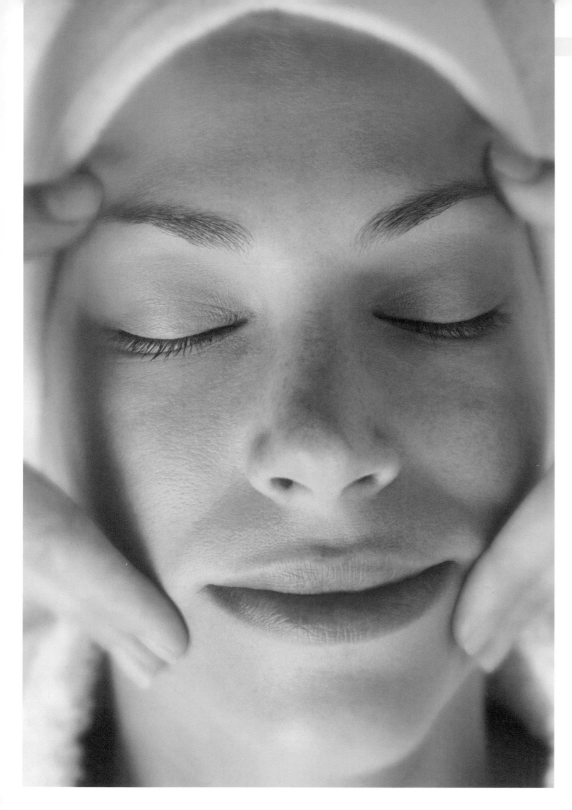

move lymph around the body. Massage directly assists lymphatic drainage by pushing lymph out of muscles and other cells and on toward the collecting nodes, speeding up the removal of waste products and toxins.

Soothing effleurage can reduce blood pressure by calming the body and reducing the cardiac output (the amount of blood forced out of the heart per minute). It also reduces peripheral resistance caused when contracted and tight muscles prevent blood from flowing freely.

Massage removes dead skin cells, allowing sweat glands, hair follicles, and sebaceous glands to be free of obstruction and so work more effectively. The blood supply to the skin is stimulated by massage, taking fresh nutrients to feed the skin. The skin also benefits from the vitamins and minerals found in massage oils.

above: Facial massage removes dead skin cells and stimulates blood flow, reinvigorating the face and relieving stress.

massage: the antidote to stress

Few people in the West are able to escape the trappings of modern living and the stresses that accompany them. Urban life causes us to rush and presents us with a constant onslaught of emotions to deal with, from other people's negativity to alarming news stories in the media. The environment constantly bombards us with noise and pollution. At work we may be exposed to sick-building syndrome and radiation from electrical equipment; at home we ingest chemicals in food.

On the inside, we suffer from our own high expectations and perfectionism, trying to achieve too much in too short a time and striving to please others. Fears and worries—founded and unfounded—assault our well-being, and keeping emotions pent up only adds to the stress. Day-to-day living is further complicated by life events; marriage, births, deaths, moving, divorce, losing a job, and going on vacation all take a toll on well-being.

left: In a high-stress world, something as simple as a foot roller kept under the office desk can make a significant impact, allowing you to self-massage and reduce anxiety levels.

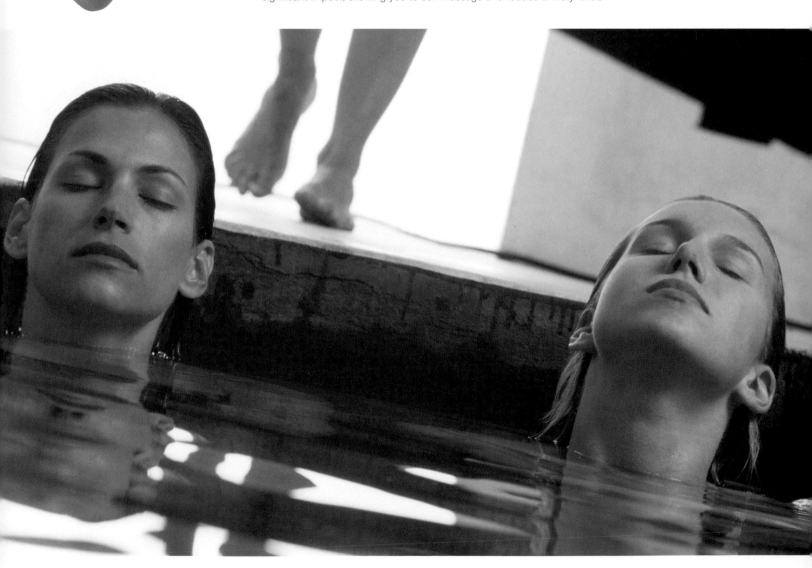

right: Meditation is an extremely useful tool in bringing calm and balance back into your life.

At work, new technology such as cell phones and e-mail mean we are often expected to take on increasing amounts of work and responsibility, meet tighter deadlines, and liaise with people far from the workplace. Expectations are often too high. In the home, increasing numbers of us juggle work, private life, and family commitments, and see the stress manifested in conflict and unhappy relationships. It is no wonder our health suffers when we are under stress.

The key problem is that modern ways of living cause the human stress response known as "fight or flight" to be activated too often and inappropriately. A cat runs out in front of the car and we slam on the brakes, experiencing palpitations; we go for an interview and suffer sweaty palms and a dry mouth; we rush around in a hurry and become tense; we have an argument and feel shaky and sick; we think of that pile of work on the desk and become anxious and exhausted.

Stress causes our muscles to tighten, literally in preparation to fight or flee. It raises our blood pressure and heart rate, causes us to breathe rapidly, and stimulates our liver to release cholesterol into our bloodstream. Definitely not good for our health!

The good news is that the stress response can be counteracted by healthy living, and, in particular, by promoting the ability to relax. Relaxation can take many forms: a warm bath, a stroll in the country, yoga, a sauna, reading a good book, meditation, breathing exercises, and, of course, massage. Through the act of relaxation, we stimulate a part of the brain, the parasympathetic nervous system, that slows the heart rate and breathing, lowers blood pressure, and stimulates the digestive and immune systems.

Massage can be one of the most effective ways to relax. It helps us switch off that nagging voice inside the head and unwind from overwork, rushing, and worries that compound. It encourages easy and deep breathing, eases the tension out of muscles, allows the heart rate to slow and blood pressure to lower, and, perhaps above all, allows us purely and simply just to be.

left: Taking time out for a swim or a day at a health spa is an important part of managing your lifestyle and your mental and physical health.

giving a massage

To make your massage as effective and pleasurable as possible, spend a few minutes on preparation before you start. A number of accessories, such as towels and oils, help make the massage more comfortable for you and your partner. Pay attention to these details and your massage will become a complete indulgence. Bear in mind that if the experience of your massage is wonderful, you are likely to be given one in return!

start at the beginning

Begin massage with an attitude of wonder and awe, curiosity and willingness. Know that there are no rights or wrongs and that by offering care and attention, you can only do right. Ask your recipient for feedback about what feels great and what you can improve on. Understand that each person is unique, with different sensitivities and varying thresholds for receiving pressure. Appreciate also that over time and with repetition, your partner's body will become more and more addicted to your intoxicating strokes, becoming able to tolerate, accept, and, finally, welcome stronger pressure.

create a sacred space

Find a quiet room with enough space for your partner to lie comfortably and for you to be able to move around his or her body. Make sure the room is warm, possibly warmer than feels comfortable, as people often become quite chilled as they relax and the body systems slow. Ensure also that the room is quiet and free from distraction: the answering machine is on with the volume turned down, the dog has been fed, the television is off, and the children are being entertained elsewhere.

To keep your partner warm, cover him or her with towels and only uncover parts of the body you are working on. Towels also protect clothing from the oil you use, which can stain. To make your partner feel really pampered, warm the towels in the dryer until you are ready to begin the massage.

To enhance the atmosphere, subdue the lighting or even give the massage by candlelight. You may wish to perfume the air with some essential oils: place five to six drops of oil in the water bowl of an oil

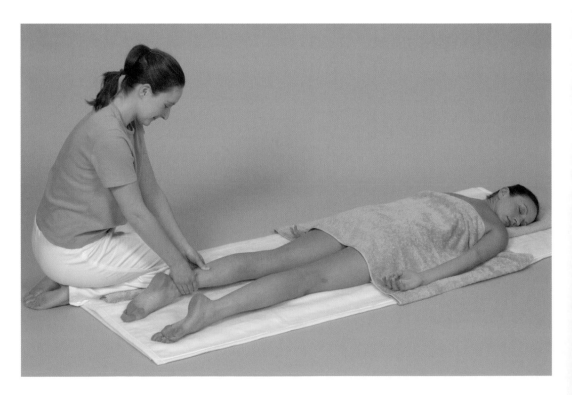

right: It is often best to position your partner on a yoga mat covered by blankets or towels on the floor. This provides enough support and allows you room to maneuver as a therapist.

burner half an hour before you start the massage. Indulge all the senses by accompanying the treatment with some carefully selected relaxing music. Compilation tapes especially for relaxation and massage are available in New Age and health stores.

prepare yourself

Before you start to make the strokes, prepare yourself to ensure that you are in the right state of mind to give the most caring and loving treatment possible. If you are relaxed and centered and have thoughts of nurturing and caring, you will be giving the greatest gift to your partner through your hands.

massage tools

The best place to give a treatment is on the floor, provided your back and knees are fit and healthy. A bed is usually too soft and a little too low to give a massage treatment, but may be used if preferred. To soften the floor, place a quilt, mattress, or futon over the area on which you will be working. You might like to use an electric blanket beneath your partner.

Keep a number of different-sized cushions, pillows, or bolsters at hand, and possibly a kneeling pad (available from gardening stores) for your knees.

You will need a large supply of big, fluffy towels to cover parts of your partner's body not being massaged. Some people become so chilled that they require a blanket: place it over the towels.

When massaging with oils, take care to avoid spills—especially on carpet where it will cause stains. Use plastic bottles with a flip top to dispense oil with little risk of spilling. You can purchase them from health stores and beauty suppliers.

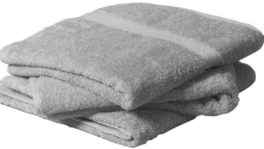

below: Make sure you have plenty of clean towels on hand for a massage. They are soft to the touch, keep your partner warm, and protect his or her modesty.

general guidelines

Preparation
- Have short, clean fingernails.
- Remove jewelry from yourself and your partner.
- Keep the room warm and free from distractions.
- Wear loose, comfortable clothes in which you can move freely.

Giving the massage
- Treat the person you are massaging with tender, loving care.
- Keep your hands in contact with your partner as much as possible as you work on each body part.
- Perform the massage slowly and in a rhythmic, flowing manner for maximum relaxation.
- Make the massage continuous and flowing; the end of one technique or repetition should flow into the beginning of the next.
- When massaging limbs, perform all the techniques on one limb before moving on to massage the other.
- Focus on the quality of your massage rather than on chatting.
- Ask for feedback about the level of pressure and the comfort and effectiveness of your techniques.
- Never put pressure on bones or joints.
- After deep massage, soothe the area with effleurage (page 44).

- With stroking techniques, the emphasis of pressure is toward the heart.
- Repeat the technique several times. It is the repetition over and over that hypnotizes the body into relaxation.

Looking after yourself
- Adopt a rocking movement of your body to assist you.
- Use your body weight rather than strength to apply pressure.
- Focus on your breathing, ensuring that you breathe slowly and as deeply as possible.
- Every now and then, take your attention back to yourself to check that you are comfortable, still relaxed, and not holding yourself in an awkward position.

After the massage
- Encourage your recipient to get up from the massage slowly in order to prevent any lightheadedness.
- Ask your partner to drink plenty of fresh water to flush away any waste products.
- Warn your partner that he or she may ache a little after the manipulations of the massage.

positioning yourself and your partner

It is important to be as comfortable as possible when giving a massage: this affects the quality of your treatment. It also helps prevent you from straining your back or hurting your knees—injuring yourself in this way could discourage you from ever giving another massage! The comfort of the recipient is paramount to a relaxing massage. In a fully supported position your partner will be able to relax totally and let go of tension.

positioning yourself

kneeling: For some strokes, a kneeling position is fine. You may prefer to work on a gardener's kneeling pad or on a pillow to take pressure off your knees and help you kneel for longer.

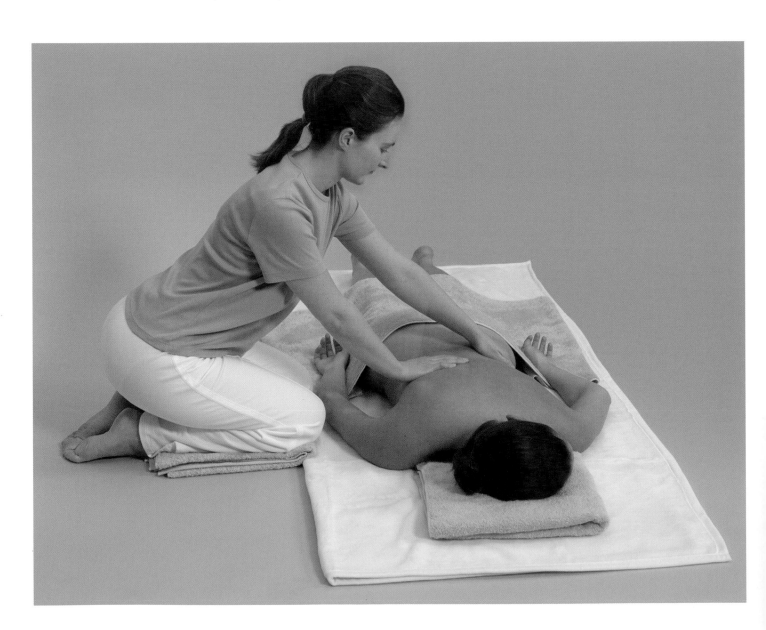

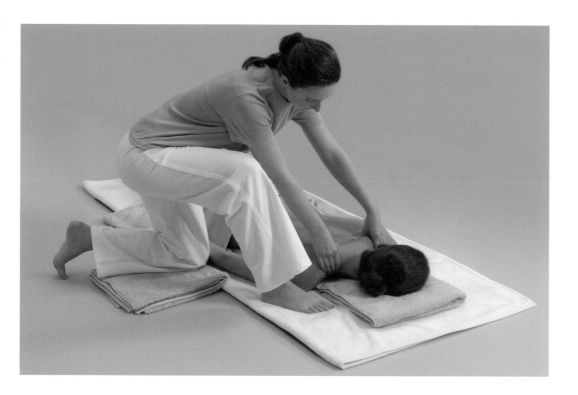

half-kneeling: Kneeling can make the knees ache and is not always the best position for massage, as it doesn't allow you to use your body weight effectively or to achieve a full range of movement. A half-kneeling position is usually preferable. From this position you can sway from side to side and forward to back to keep your massage techniques fluid and flowing. Practice these body movements before you begin the massage. From this elevated position you will also be able to lean over your partner and use the weight of your body to increase the pressure behind the techniques.

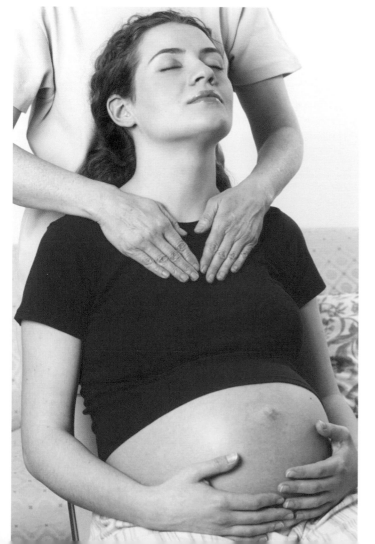

right: Pregnant women can enjoy great benefits from the muscular relief of massage, some of which can be applied while seated.

positioning your partner

lying prone: When working on the back and back of the legs, ask your partner to lie on his or her front. Carefully positioned pillows or cushions can make lying on the floor more comfortable. Experiment by placing a small cushion beneath the abdomen and/or chest, another under the head, and one under the feet. Or try a rolled-up towel or bolster. If comfortable, the best position for your partners' arms is by their sides. If your partner is pregnant, has a back problem, or is elderly, a prone position may not be comfortable and you might like to try a seated back massage instead (page 172).

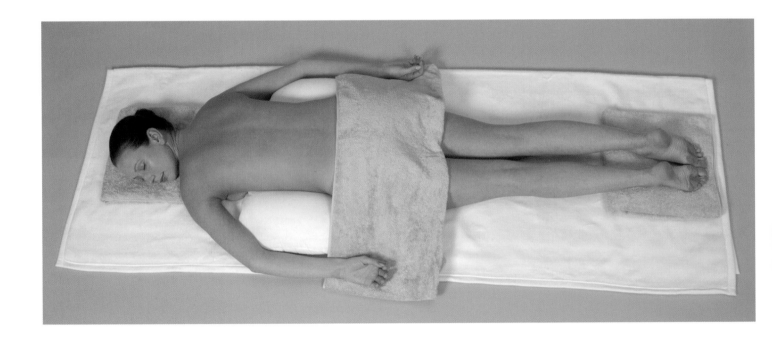

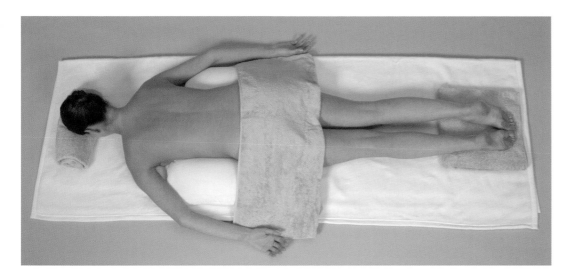

Some people find lying with their head turned to one side creates stiffness in the neck. To help keep the spine and back in alignment, place a cushion or rolled up towel under the forehead so they can relax with their head facing straight down. Make sure there is enough room for their nose—you may need two cushions! A cushion under the abdomen can offer support to someone with a lower-back problem.

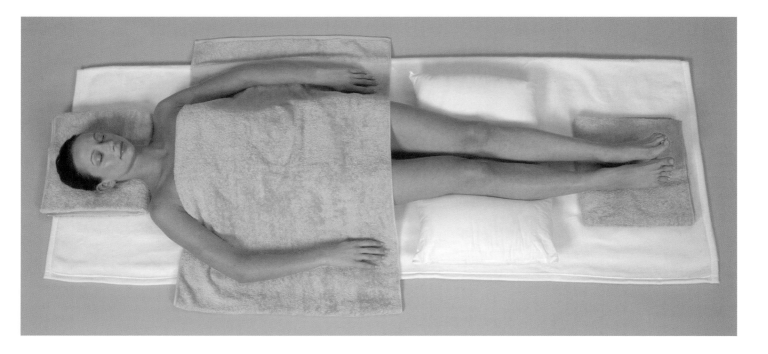

lying supine: For massaging the rest of the body, ask your partner to lie on his or her back. Those with a lower-back problem should take the pressure off the back by bending the knees, or you can place a bolster or pillow under the knees. Some people will be more comfortable with a pillow beneath the head as well. It is not advisable for heavily pregnant women to lie supine: prop them up with several pillows or work with the woman on her side (page 161).

massage basics

A massage once a day would not be often enough in my book. Give massage as often as you can, performing it slowly to make it truly relaxing. Each technique is repeated over and over again, to hypnotize the body into a state of deep relaxation. Bearing in mind the following essentials will help you work toward this ideal.

movement

Massage can be likened to a dance or to meditation in motion, in which the gentle and rhythmic swaying of your body as you perform the massage strokes transports you and your partner into a state of complete relaxation. You will find that physical strength is not necessary if you use your body weight to lean into the techniques to create pressure and if you allow your body movement as you lean away from the body to assist you in manipulating muscle away from bone.

body weight

If you try to use strength alone to give your massage techniques depth, you will soon tire. It is far better to use your own body weight to lean into the stroke. When adding weight to a stroke in this way, build up slowly and ask your partner for feedback as to how much depth he or she can tolerate. Some people enjoy a really deep massage, while others prefer a light touch. It is better to start lightly and build up, rather than be heavy-handed to the point of hurting. When applying effleurage, you may be able to use much more body weight.

pressure and pleasurable pain

In order for massage techniques to be effective, it is important to use some pressure; otherwise we are simply tickling. Everyone has their own pain threshold, and the giving and receiving of massage is supposed to be a pleasure. However, there is a pleasurable pain in massage when the stroke just hits the spot and the therapeutic benefits feel so great that the hurt becomes a relief. Talk to your partner about his or her preferences and be willing to experiment. It is common for the skin to turn red after pressure work; this is a good sign as long as the skin does not feel sore.

pace and repetition

Massage is usually done slowly to make it truly relaxing. Each technique is repeated over and over again, to hypnotize the body into a state of deep relaxation.

frequency

Regular massage is the key. Give a massage every day if you can.

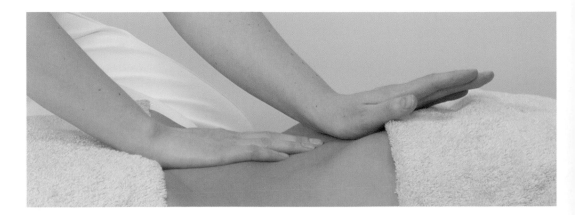

massage oils

Oil allows your hands to slip over your partner's skin during massage without causing friction, dragging, or slipping. Good-quality, unrefined, cold-pressed, additive-free vegetable oils are the most suitable oils for massage. It is well known that oils such as olive oil form part of a healthy diet; likewise if applied to the body, vegetable oils not only allow your massage movements to flow smoothly, they nourish the skin from the outside.

Choose the best-quality oils you can afford and store them somewhere cool and dark with the lids on tightly: exposure to light, heat, and oxygen causes oils to go rancid. To help keep oil fresh, add a few drops of wheat-germ oil to the bottle. As well as increasing the shelf life of the oil, this boosts its vitamin E content. The most suitable oils for massage include sweet almond, apricot kernel, avocado, safflower, and sunflower oil. Allergies (to nut oils, among others) seem to be on the increase, so do a patch test by rubbing a drop of oil on the inside of the elbow or wrist of the massage recipient before using a new oil. A rash usually appears within twenty-four hours if the skin reacts; if it does, try another oil.

below: Sunflower oil can be found in most kitchens and is ideal as a massage oil.

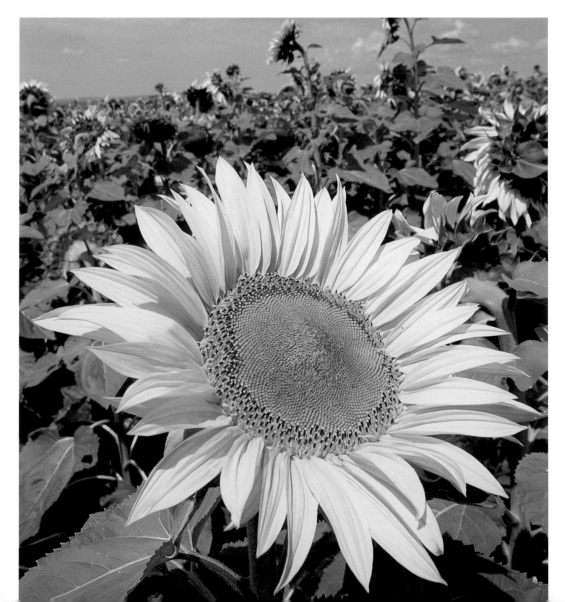

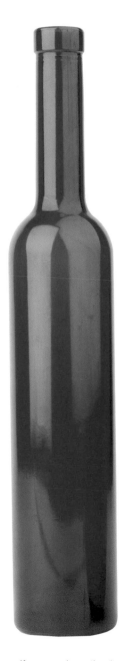

above: If you are investing in good-quality massage oils, it is best to keep them in dark-colored bottles to preserve them.

how to use oil

1. Decant some oil into a plastic bottle with a flip top to avoid spills. Pour a little oil into the palm of one hand (pouring oil directly onto your partner may give him or her a shock). Keep the back of your hand resting on the skin as you pour.

2. Warm the oil between your hands before applying it to your partner's skin, without breaking contact with your partner's body.

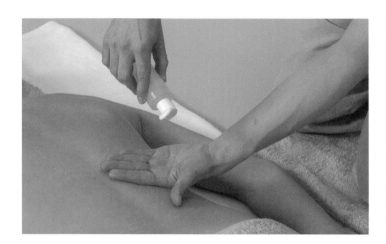

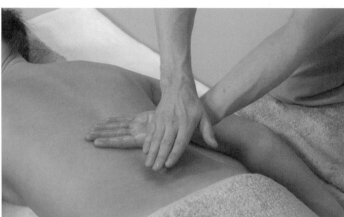

3. Spread the oil over your partner's skin using large, sweeping strokes. Keep the bottle within reach as you massage in case the oil is quickly absorbed and you need to apply more. Take care not to use too much oil, though: start using about a tablespoon at a time on each of the different areas of the body, adding more as you need it.

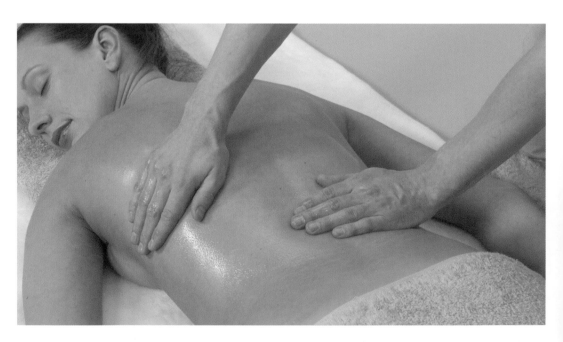

types of oil

Sweet almond oil: Popular for massage, as it nourishes the skin and is easily but not too quickly absorbed. For facial massage, dilute with a lighter oil such as apricot kernel if your partner finds it a little too greasy. Unrefined sweet almond oil can help relieve the symptoms of eczema, either by direct application to the skin or by adding to the bath.

Apricot kernel oil: Lighter and more expensive than almond oil, it's a good facial massage oil either in its pure form or blended with another oil such as sweet almond. This has a stronger aroma than some oils, but its gentle nature makes it useful for dry, sensitive, and more mature skins.

Evening primrose oil: Because of its high levels of GLA (gamma linoleic acid), evening primrose oil is useful in facial oil blends, especially any that are designed to treat dry or more mature complexions.

Jojoba: A liquid wax with a very light texture. A good oil for the face, nourishing combination or oily skin, and especially good for acne-prone skin. This is one of the more expensive oils.

Olive oil: A fairly sticky oil, which is good to use on severely dehydrated skin, chapped hands, or sore and inflamed skin. Cold-pressed virgin olive oils are available in supermarkets, but the more viscous nature and pungent smell of the oil means that it is often mixed with equal parts of a lighter oil, such as sweet almond, for massage.

Sunflower oil: Another oil available in supermarkets that makes an excellent moisturizer and massage oil. It has little smell and is a light-textured oil, suitable for blending with other oils for massage. It is particularly suitable for use with babies.

above: Apricot oil is particularly suitable for facial massages.

Wheat-germ oil: The richest natural source of vitamin E, this can be added to all oil blends to increase their shelf life by delaying rancidity. Straight wheat-germ oil is good for more mature skins and can speed the healing of scar tissue; it is especially good on skin that has been overexposed to sunlight. By itself, wheat-germ oil is a little heavy for massage, but it can be mixed successfully with lighter oils to achieve a more suitable consistency.

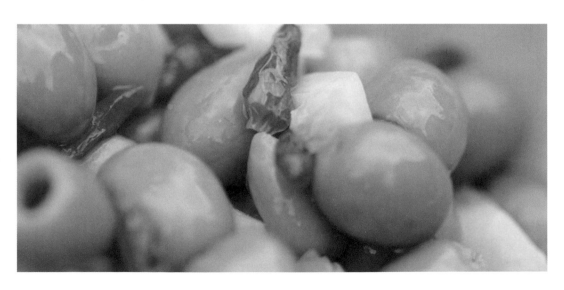

left: Olive oil is extremely good for dehydrated skin.

massage and the senses

We encounter the world through our senses, relying on the ability to smell, feel, hear, taste, and see for our daily safety and well-being. We may see or hear danger, smell a fire, and depend on touch to function at the most basic level every day, often without being aware of it—the touch of a chair against the buttocks, for instance, informs us that it is safe to sit down.

In addition to these functional attributes, the senses are vital for mental, emotional, and spiritual well-being. In China, it is believed that the senses are united with the universe. They are the gateway to all that happens and the windows of our whole being. It is well known that each molecule, every atom of the universe is in constant vibration, vibrating at its own frequency and wavelength. The vibrations of sound, color, smell, taste, heat, and light enter our bodies constantly through each of the senses. We can use all these media to enhance massage treatments and help the body restore the balance of mind, body, and spirit. Try some of the tips that follow.

smell

A penetrating aroma cultivates all the senses. It can titillate the taste buds and act as an anchor for memory. The memory center plays a vital role in emotional responses.
- Ensure the air is clean and pure by using an ionizer or humidifier.
- Place herb pillows under your partner's head.
- Use cut flowers to bring invigorating energy and perfume to the room (clear glass vases in curved shapes add tranquil qi energy).
- Use essential oils in an oil burner.

sound

Pleasing sounds encourage relaxation and are an important link with nature. Sounds vibrate the air, stimulating the flow of qi energy. Music is such an effective way to change moods and create an atmosphere that it makes a powerful and important tool to accompany massage. Calming, hauntingly evocative music opens body and soul to receive the benefits of powerful massage.
- Play music that incorporates natural sounds, such as birdsong, leaves rustling, babbling brooks, and waves.
- Bring healing sounds into the room with an indoor waterfall and wind chimes.
- Be aware that silence, too, is just as important for physical and emotional health.

sight

Clear, natural light from the sun raises the spirits and encourages health and well-being through the pineal gland. Light is energy in its truest form. Light and color create atmosphere. Combined, they have the ability to dazzle or enhance, dim or brighten.
- To increase light, fill the room with mirrors, crystals, and candles (float them in water).
- Use full-spectrum daylight bulbs.
- Receive a massage in a warm, sun-bathed room and sense how delicious it feels.

  Color affects us emotionally, physically, and spiritually. It stimulates the senses by encouraging relaxation or activity. Choose the color of towels and accessories with care, and ask your partner to contemplate a color during the massage. Every color is linked with key characteristics.

BLUE: harmony, peace
VIOLET: sensitivity, the royal color
RED: warmth, vitality
ORANGE: invigoration, warmth
YELLOW: uplifting joy
GREEN: hope, the color of nature

taste

The energy of all five senses should be in harmony. To bring the sense of taste into your treatment, offer your partner an herbal tea or juice before and after massage.

touch

Quality touch is important for mental, emotional, physical, and spiritual well-being. To enhance the touch of your hands, use warm, fluffy towels and perhaps an electric blanket. Covering your partner with a blanket creates a sense of weight and reassurance over the body.

nature

Spending time outdoors is an effective way to soothe and heal the mind. Bring nature into the treatment room with freshly cut flowers, natural sunlight, and the sounds of birds and water.

stillness and silence

In the modern world we simply do not have enough stillness and silence. Massage is an ideal time to redress the balance. For some or all of your massage, do it in silence without music or talking. It can really feel sacred. Laying still hands on your companion for a while can be deeply relaxing.

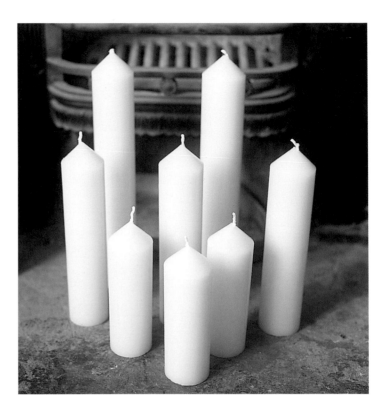

above: Have plenty of candles on hand when setting up your massage environment, as they help create a positive and calming mood.

below: Take your inspiration from the colors and moods of the natural world. Too often, modern life excludes the calming influence of nature.

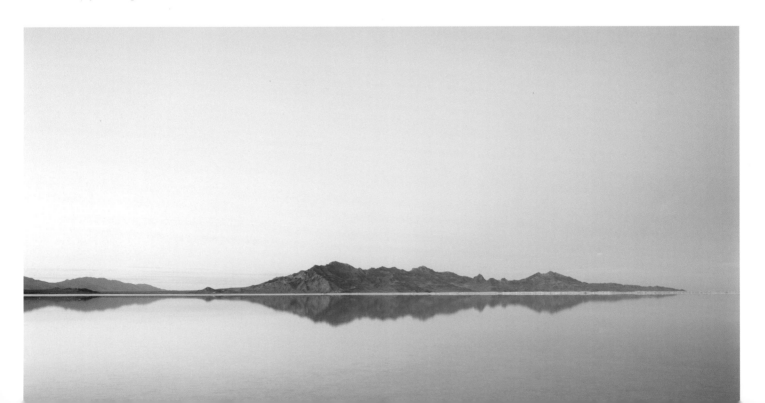

massage as ritual

Massage is a two-way flow of touch and response—a mutual exchange of energy. The hands, that both give and receive, and the skin are the instruments of communication. Through your hands, you perceive and discover the uniqueness of the person you are touching. Through the skin, your massage partner receives the gift of your touch, caring contact, and movement. In a sense, the terms "giver" and "receiver" are deceptive, since any form of touch therapy is a matter of sharing.

For the healing power of touch to be transmitted, both partners must understand their roles in the exchange. Use some of the energy work ideas on pages 34–37 to encourage both partners to learn how to give and to be receptive—the receiver giving trust and surrendering to the giver; the giver being open and sensitive to the needs of the receiver.

right: The seven chakras seen here can be stimulated to heighten senses and awareness.

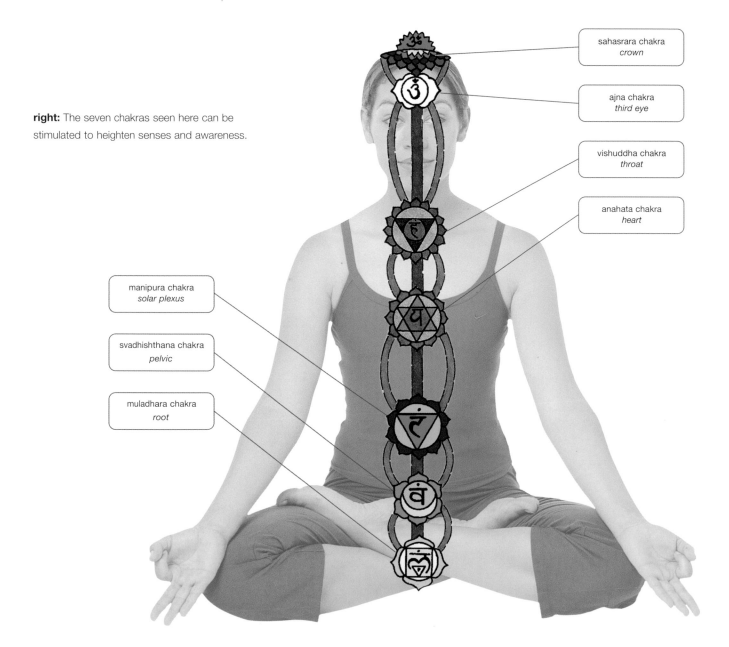

sahasrara chakra
crown

ajna chakra
third eye

vishuddha chakra
throat

anahata chakra
heart

manipura chakra
solar plexus

svadhishthana chakra
pelvic

muladhara chakra
root

massage as meditation

At its highest level, massage can be a form of meditation, with both participants present in the moment, each focused on the point of contact between them. As part of the massage, ensure you both give permission and thanks for the massage by building an element of ritual into the treatment.

healing energy

Many cultures believe that the body is more than a collection of parts. They acknowledge an essential inner energy that constantly flows through the body from conception, throughout life, and perhaps into the afterlife. This energy is known in China as *qi*, in India as *prana*, and in Tibet as *lung*. Although the concept seems alien to many modern Western minds, it was once accepted in Europe too. The second-century physician Galen called the body's energy *pneuma*, and medical alchemists used the term "vital fluid." According to all these systems, energy permeates the physical body—the organs, muscles, bones, and glands—but also reaches beyond the physical to the mental and spiritual planes. Illness is believed to begin not when symptoms show, but when the energy flow is first disrupted. The balance of energy can be deeply affected by stress, shock, or emotional factors. Good health depends on a smooth, steady flow of energy, which requires mental, spiritual, and physical balance.

The key concept of Traditional Chinese Medicine is the understanding that "rivers of energy" known as "meridians" run throughout the body. In the Indian approach, the body's energy is thought to generate from and be regulated by a chakra system, chakras being visualized as spinning wheels of energy running down the center of the body. The third-body energy system was developed in the West and is used by healers and clairvoyants in Europe and the United States. It is similar to the Indian chakra system in that layers of energy are believed to surround the body. These layers are linked to the chakras and form an aura, and successive layers emit different vibrations of energy. Energy is thought to move between people via thought and meditation, and the energy of every person is considered to affect, directly or indirectly, the energy of every other person in the world. We can all see how affected we are by the atmosphere created by the energy of our partners, parents, children, or close friends, and watch how our responses change whenever those around us are happy, excited, or depressed.

Healing through touch or thought may be the oldest form of energy medicine. It was known to the Egyptians and Greeks. Massage therapists incorporate healing in their work by transmitting energy from one person to another through hands. This transmission triggers the receiver's capacity for self-healing.

your energy force

The body's energy is a subtle, yet powerful force and one that is crucial to physical and spiritual well-being. Luckily, we do not always have to be conscious of it or tending to it. Looking after the body's energy is like breathing—we do it constantly, regularly, and without thinking. However, by nurturing your energy, you can improve its quality and greatly benefit vitality. This in turn gives greater resistance to fight illness. All matter is made of energy. It permeates every realm of existence, unifying the cosmos and uniting every atom in the body. It is what makes the heart beat and eyes shine. The sun gives energy to all living things on earth, and we all respond to changes in its power. The moon is another powerful force, influencing both the tides and women's menstrual cycles.

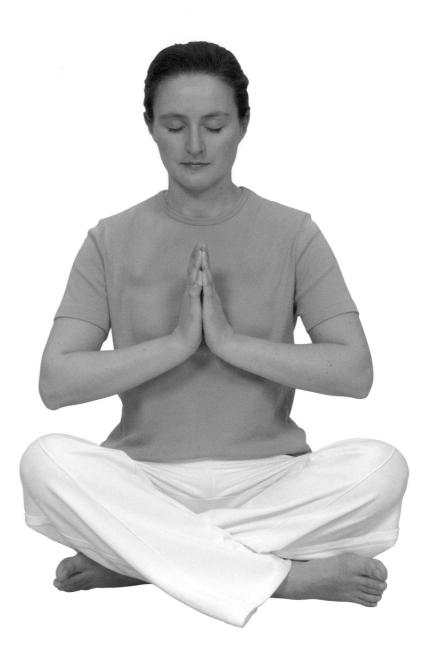

above: Use the heart salutation
to prepare yourself for giving a
massage.

energy bath

There is a subtle energetic link between every living thing on the planet. Everyone is part of this delicate, life-giving balance, and we can all benefit by drawing energy from the natural world. Spend time in natural places to absorb their energy: historic sights, waterfalls, the huge expanse of the sea, mountain peaks, ancient forests, or the sunshine of your own yard. Anyone who has looked up at the clear blue sky on a fresh spring morning or leaned back in a deck chair to close their eyes and soak up the heat of a summer afternoon will testify to the energizing qualities of the natural world.

heart salutation

The heart salutation is a beautiful way to start and finish a massage. Place your hands in a prayer position, palms touching, thumbs against the center of your chest. This is an acupressure point known as the "sea of tranquility," which centers and balances. Breathe deeply, close your eyes, and make a prayer or a wish or set an intention for the person you are with.

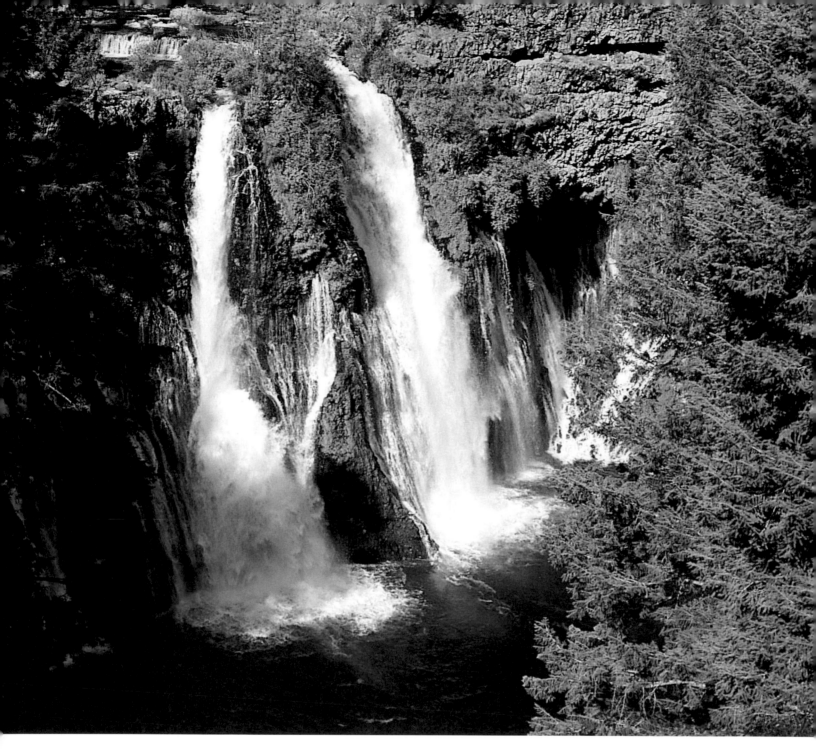

grounding and centering

Before giving a massage, spend a few minutes centering yourself. Centering is a way of focusing, of gathering your energy into a point so that you can channel it more easily. It comprises a state of balance, quietness, strength, and presence in the moment. More specifically, centering means focusing on the *hara*, the center of energy in the abdomen. *Hara* is the Japanese word for the belly or abdomen. Commonly regarded as the "earth" center, it allows for the energy from the earth to be gathered up into the pelvis, then relayed out via the arms and hands. It is our center of gravity, equilibrium, and stability; the nucleus of our physical and psychic powers.

For any form of massage, being centered in the hara is of prime importance, for it enables you to be flexible yet resilient, to work with intuition rather than the mind. When your energy is channeled, you need less muscle power and can give a massage without becoming tired or drained. Being centered also entails correct posture—spine erect and neck and shoulders relaxed—and remaining grounded, aware of your contact with the earth through your legs and feet.

above: Recordings of sounds from nature, such as waterfalls, can be used to help create a calming environment.

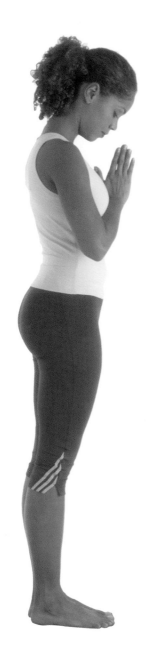

To center yourself, stand upright, close your eyes, and direct your attention inward. Feel the strong foundation of your feet as they maintain contact with the floor. From this firm base, allow your spine to float gently upward without any strain. Let go of any tension in your shoulders, neck, and face. Now focus on the breath, allowing it to find its own rhythm. Imagine that as you inhale, your breath fills your lower abdomen, or hara. After a few breaths, begin to visualize that as you exhale, your breath flows up your torso from the hara, through your shoulders, down your arms, and out of your hands. Visualize the breath as a stream of energy or white light, flowing up the body and out of your fingers.

attention and intention

To give a truly amazing massage, give total attention to every movement, massaging with a heightened awareness of the intention of the treatment. This could be to give massage in a loving way, to nurture, to relax the recipient, or to ease physical or emotional pain. Anything done lovingly is a spiritual act, and this is never so true as with massage.

developing qi (energy)

To get a sense of this energy it is very easy to get in touch with it within your own body.

❶ Sit or stand comfortably and begin to rub your hands together vigorously, feeling the heat being generated and continuing for as long as you can. Stop and notice how your hands are tingling.

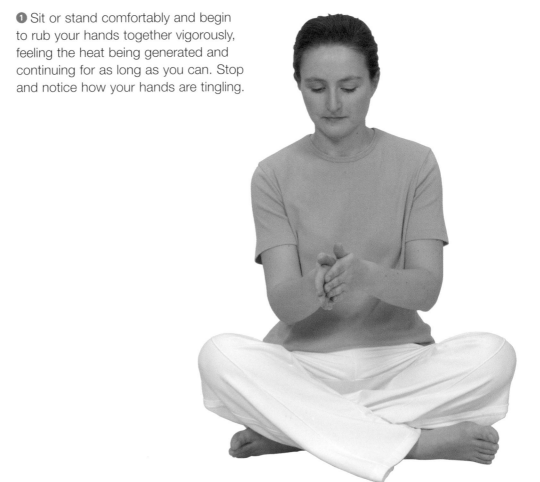

above: Prior to a massage, take a few moments to stand with your eyes closed and your focus turned inward in order to center yourself.

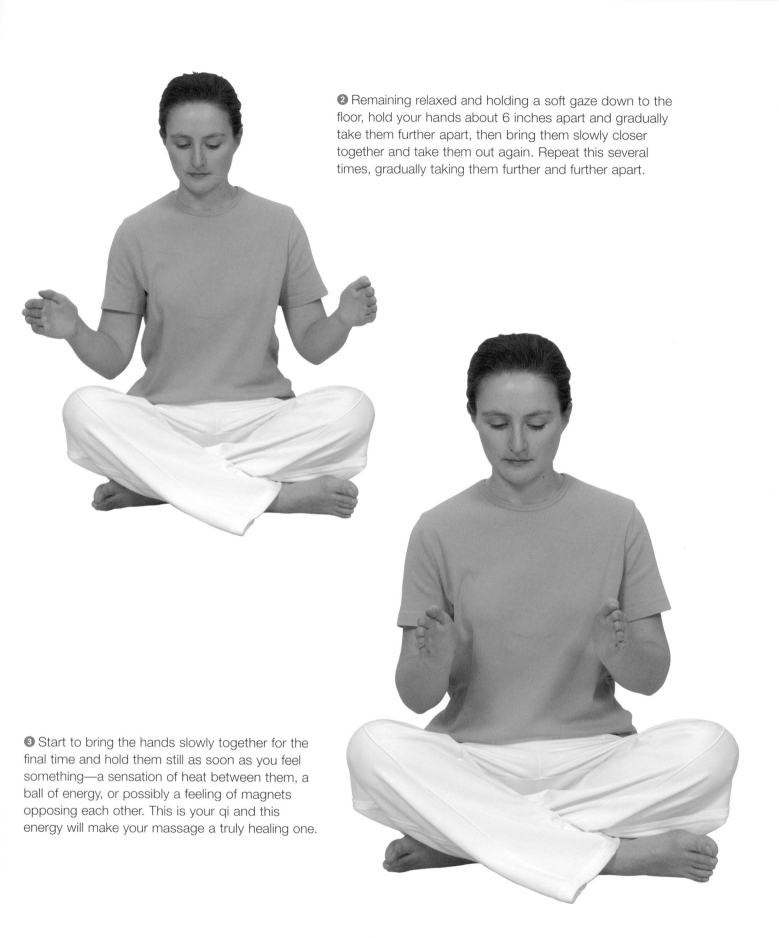

❷ Remaining relaxed and holding a soft gaze down to the floor, hold your hands about 6 inches apart and gradually take them further apart, then bring them slowly closer together and take them out again. Repeat this several times, gradually taking them further and further apart.

❸ Start to bring the hands slowly together for the final time and hold them still as soon as you feel something—a sensation of heat between them, a ball of energy, or possibly a feeling of magnets opposing each other. This is your qi and this energy will make your massage a truly healing one.

safety guidelines

On the whole, massage is a very safe therapy. However, in some situations it is not advisable to massage. There is not enough room in this book to cover all the diseases and disorders of the human body, but the most common contraindications for massage are set out here. If, for any reason, you are not sure whether massage is suitable for your partner, don't do it. It is always advisable to consult a medical practitioner before massaging if you have any doubts.

Varicose veins and thrombosis

Never massage with any pressure over a varicose vein (usually found in the legs) or below it. Blood clots may be attached to the vein wall; pressure could dislodge them, freeing the clot to travel in the blood stream to the heart or brain and cause serious injury, such as a stroke. If you are in any doubt as to whether a vein is varicose, avoid the area and massage another part of the body. Light effleurage is often permissible. For people with a history of deep vein thrombosis (blood clots), obtain permission from their doctor before giving a massage.

Heart conditions

People with conditions such as angina can benefit enormously from the relaxation massage provides and also the boosted circulation. As massage stimulates the flow of blood around the body and possibly away from the heart; however, it may be too much for a tired, weak heart to cope with. Check with the client's doctor before giving a massage.

Inflammation

Deep massage worsens any type of inflammation, whether an inflamed injury, irritable bowels, or an inflamed arthritic joint. Indications of inflammation include heat, pain or discomfort, swelling, and redness. Light, gentle stroking, however, may offer some relief and comfort. Treat undiagnosed inflammation under the skin (any unusual lump or bump) with caution. It may indicate a cyst that might burst or, more worryingly, a cancerous growth.

Scar tissue

Skin heals quickly over the site of a scar, but underlying tissue may take months or longer to heal and can remain sensitive for years. Gentle effleurage encourages fresh blood to the area and helps the healing process, but avoid firmer strokes, which could cause trauma to an already traumatized area.

High temperature

Massage may increase the temperature of someone with a fever. Refrain from massage until the recipient is fully well.

Skin problems

People with skin problems, such as eczema and psoriasis, can benefit greatly from massage. Massage oil could possibly irritate the condition, so do a small test patch by rubbing a drop of the oil you plan to use on the inside of the recipient's wrist or elbow twenty-four hours before the massage to check for reactions. Never massage over the skin lesions known as Kaposi's sarcoma, often found in people with AIDS.

Cuts, bruises, and areas of pain

It makes sense to avoid working over cuts and bruises that could be painful, and it is advisable to cover cuts with a bandage on your or your partner's skin to avoid any cross infection. Avoid areas of pain, although a very light stroking may be soothing.

Injuries and fractures

I do not massage any recent injuries and advise that you leave the treatment of injury to qualified health professionals.

Seriously ill with diabetes

If someone's diabetes is making them very ill and their circulation is being affected, do not massage.

Cancer

One school of thought postulates that massage can spread cancer through the lymphatic system. While this remains unproven and there is much evidence to dispute the theory, it is a good idea to obtain permission from a doctor before massaging people with cancer.

Pregnancy and full stomach

During the first three months of pregnancy, do not massage with any pressure on the abdomen and lower back: this is the most common time period for miscarriage, and massage can stimulate contractions. See also the specific advice on page 158. During the first two or three days of menstruation, massage on the abdomen and lower back may make bleeding heavier; check your partner's preference before giving a massage. Avoid massaging if someone has just eaten, as the massage could make them feel nauseated.

Infections

It is common sense to avoid touching anything infectious such as athlete's foot and also not to treat someone if they have a contagious disease such as chicken pox.

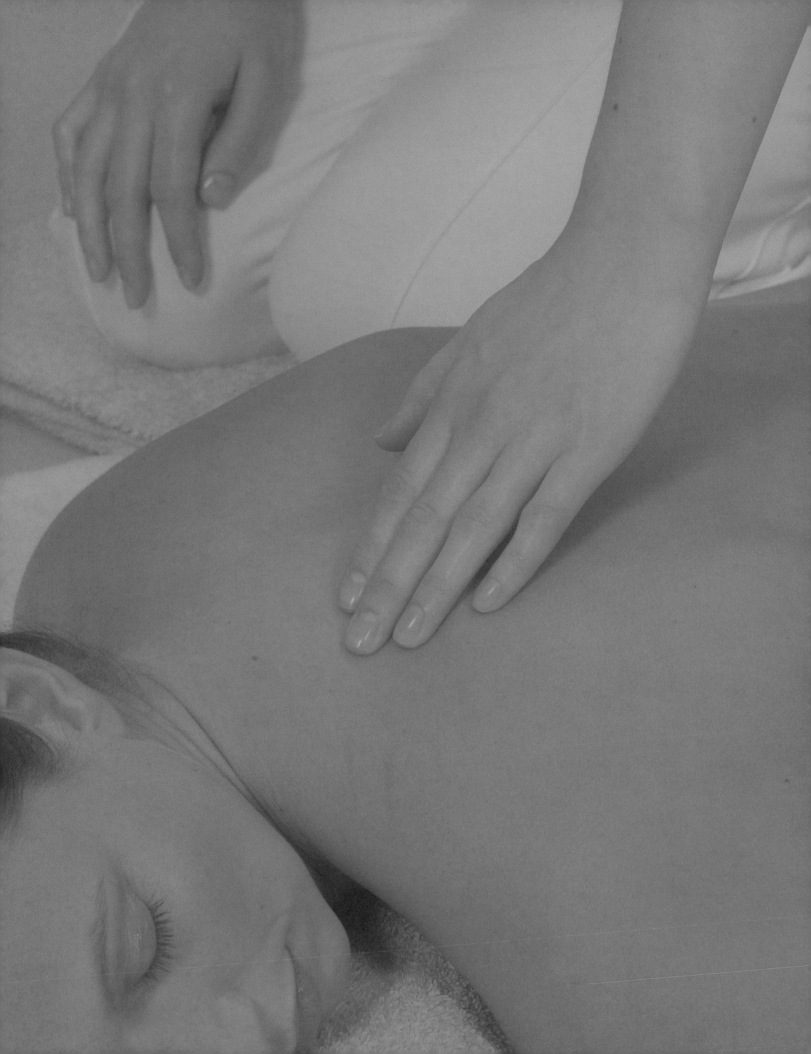

massage fundamentals

This chapter introduces some of the key techniques that make up the foundations of Swedish massage. Spend some time familiarizing yourself with these techniques and you will be able to apply them to most parts of the body. Remember that if you work slowly and with care, and avoid pressure on the joints and bones, it is fine to experiment with the strokes, asking the recipient for feedback as you go.

starting and finishing a massage

As part of the ritual of massage, it is important to start and finish with lots of care and attention and to set the scene well to make the treatment as caring, comforting, and nurturing as possible. Once the massage is complete, help the recipient realize that the session has come to a close by brushing down over the towels. This is a wonderful way to ensure that every part of the body has been touched if you have not had time to perform a full-body massage.

starting the massage

❶ First ground yourself, using the techniques on pages 35–36. Take some deep breaths and check whether your partner feels comfortable and is well covered with towels to keep warm.

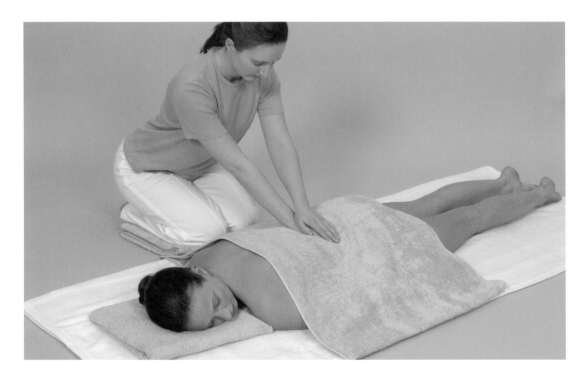

❷ To start the strokes in a pleasant way, place your hands on your partner's body and synchronize your breathing pattern with your partner's. Encourage your partner to take long, deep breaths, and let your own breathing pattern match these inhalations and exhalations for a minute or two.

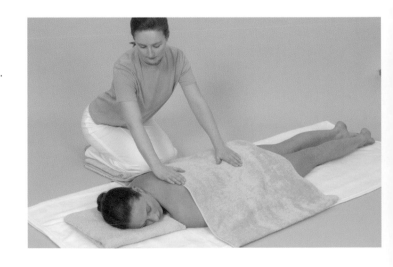

❸ Start to stroke your partner over the towel, gently and slowly. This acclimatizes your partner to your touch and induces a state of relaxation that deepens the effects of the massage.

finishing and brushing down

❶ Replace the towels to cover your partner's body, place your hands on your partner, and synchronize your breathing pattern with your partner's. Encourage your partner to take long, deep breaths, and let your own breathing pattern match these inhalations and exhalations for a minute or two.

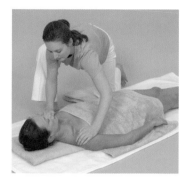 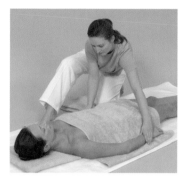

❷ If you finish the massage with your partner lying on his or her back, brush down across the towels covering the top of the chest, then down over the arms and hands. Repeat several times.

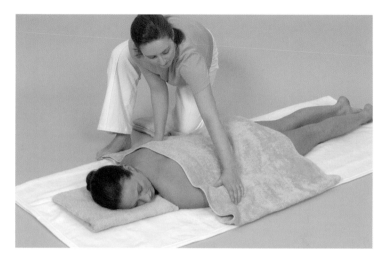

❹ If you finish the massage with your partner lying on his or her front, brush across the towels covering the top of the back and down the arms and hands. Repeat several times. Brush down the back, back of legs, and feet several times.

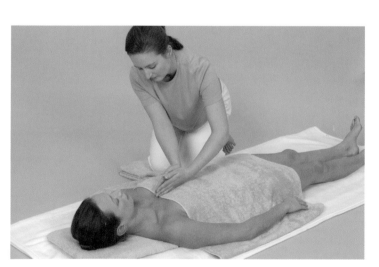

❸ With palms touching in prayer position, stroke down the center of the chest, avoiding the breasts, then flatten the hands to brush down the sides of the body and down the legs and feet. Repeat several times.

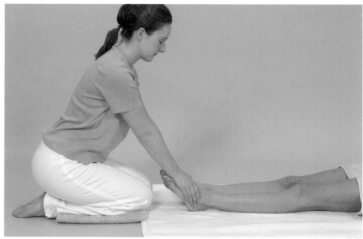

❺ Finish by holding the feet to ground the recipient. Leave your partner in peace for a few minutes, allowing time for the body to digest the effects of the massage and for your partner to come to slowly. It is likely that your partner's blood pressure will have reduced, so ensure that, when ready, he or she gets up slowly.

effleurage

These are the most fundamental massage strokes to learn: every massage in this book begins and ends with effleurage. It has a very important role in relaxing and preparing the body for deeper techniques, can soothe after deep tissue work, and is useful as a link from one technique to another or one part of the body to another. Once you are familiar with the basic techniques shown here, take a look at the respective body parts in Part 3 to learn how to apply effleurage to different areas of the body.

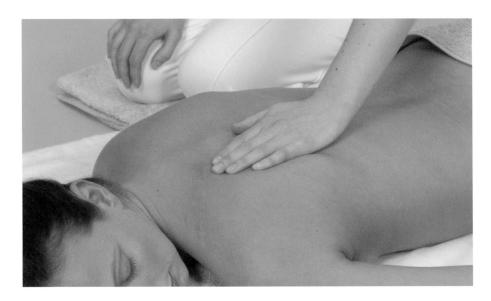

stroking
Let your hands make gentle, soothing, nurturing strokes to calm the whole area you are working, always keeping in contact with the skin as far as you can and stroking toward the heart. There is no right or wrong way to do this; see it as an opportunity to be creative and intuitive.

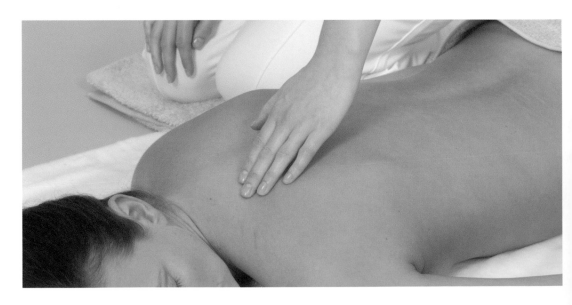

gliding
In many of the techniques that follow, you are instructed to glide your hand to get back to the start of the stroke so you can repeat the technique again. Keep the movement gentle and perform it with the fingers rather than the whole hand. Again there is no right or wrong technique, as long as you work with focus and care.

pressure

Pressure techniques are very useful for areas holding a lot of tension, for manipulating deep muscles underlying other muscles, and for working on very small muscles. These strokes are very simple to perform, but need to be applied with caution, as they can be painful—ask your partner for feedback.

CAUTION: Never apply pressure on joints.

static pressure

thumb pressure: Place your thumb on a muscle and gradually apply constant pressure by leaning in slowly using your body weight. Hold the pressure for several seconds, then release slowly.

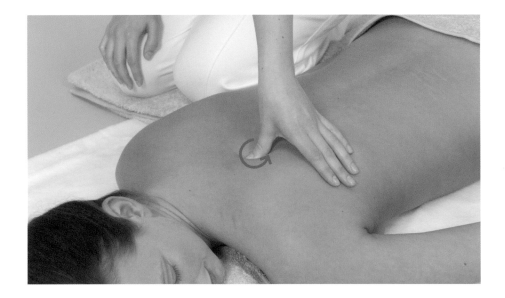

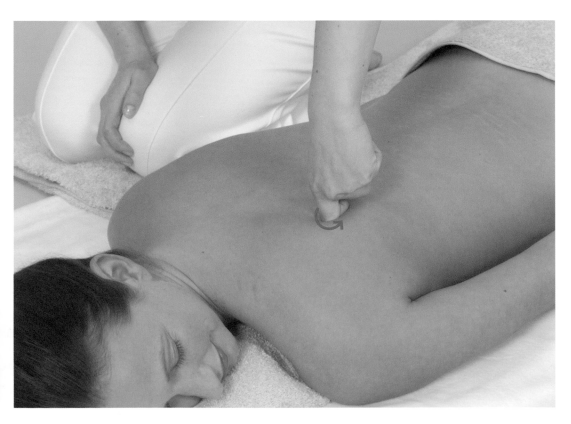

knuckle pressure: If using your thumb creates too much stress on the thumb joint, apply weight using your knuckles. Make loose fists and place the knuckles on the muscle to be worked. Very carefully apply your body weight, as described for thumb pressure.

traveling pressure

Place your thumbs side by side at the bottom of the muscle to be worked. Press into the muscle with both thumbs and glide them up the length of the muscle. Glide your hands back down slowly to repeat.

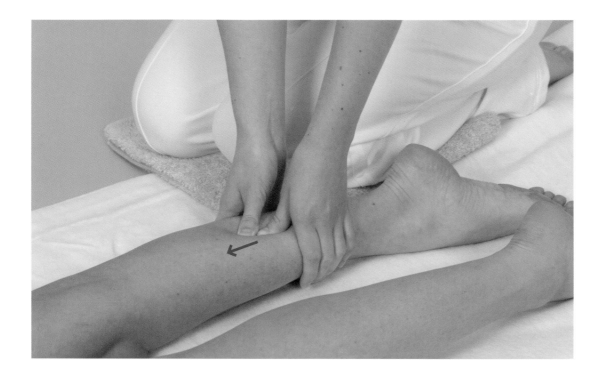

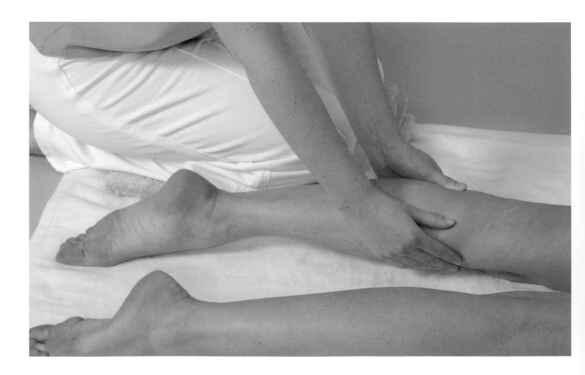

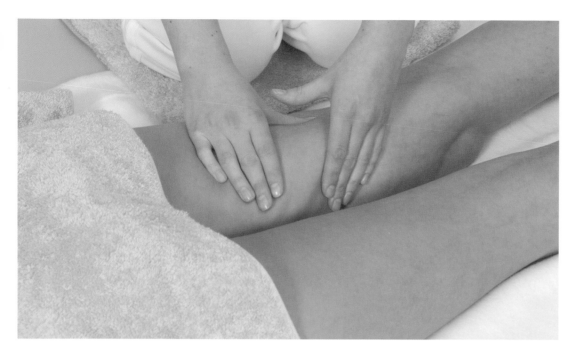

rolling pressure

❶ Position your hands near the bottom of the muscles to be worked. Push one thumb into the muscle, and exerting pressure, glide it up 1–2 inches of muscle.

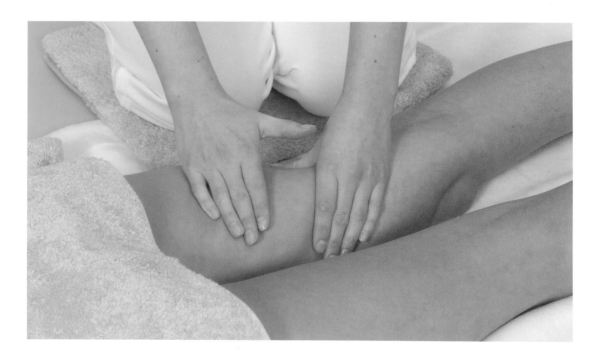

❷ Let the other thumb follow in the same way, and roll the first thumb over the top of the second one. Repeat to work gradually up the length of muscle, then glide back down to the starting position.

wringing

A squeezing and lifting movement, this technique can be used as a link between other strokes. You can vary the depth and speed of your strokes, gently kneading for a relaxing massage or working more strongly and deeply to manipulate the muscle for effective tension release.

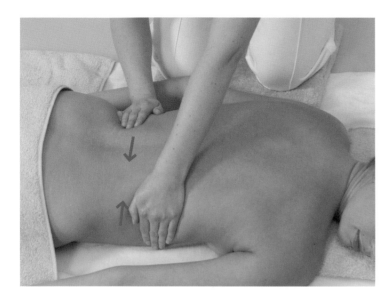

❶ Place both hands on the muscle to be worked, with fingers and thumbs pointing away from you. Glide one hand away from you and one toward you.

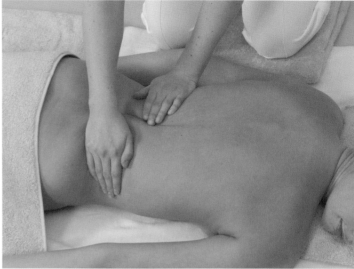

❸ Let your hands cross over so that the hand that started nearest you is furthest away and vice versa.

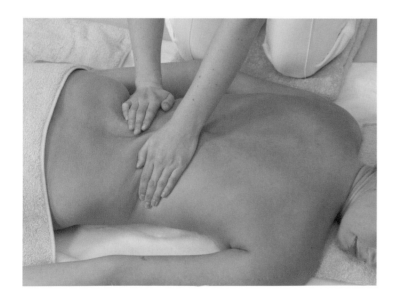

❷ Pull your hands toward each other, lifting the muscle away from the bone. To achieve a strong manipulation, lift your body weight upward to help you.

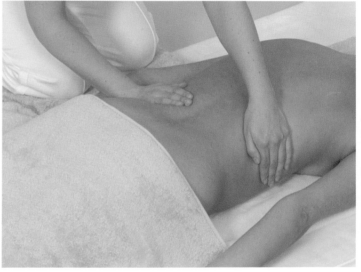

❹ Repeat, keeping as much of the palms of your hands as possible in contact with your partner's skin as you crisscross your hands all the way down the muscle.

combing and raking

Use these strokes to work any of the body's muscles more effectively once you have relaxed and prepared the area with effleurage. The pressure can be light or firm: experiment to vary the effect of the massage.

combing

❶ Lightly rest the back of your fingers on the muscle to be worked. Rest your other hand nearby. As if combing hair, use your fingers to comb the muscle from the center of the body outward.

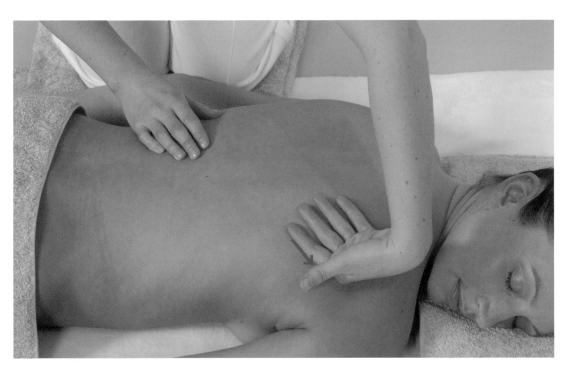

❷ When you reach the outside of the muscle, lift your hand away and return it to the starting position, ready to repeat the stroke. If working on a large muscle or large expanse of the body, gradually work along the length of the area before returning to the starting point to begin again.

raking

❶ While many of the techniques in this book are deep manipulations, it is very relaxing to receive lighter strokes such as raking. Make rakes with your hands by slightly tensing and spreading your fingers as if holding a ball.

❷ With firm pressure, pull one hand down a short area of muscle. As one hand is about to leave the body, the other hand repeats the process. Perform the technique by gradually working down the length of the muscle. The second set is started about halfway down the path of the first.

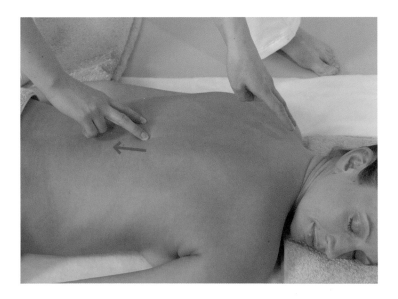

percussive techniques

Occasionally, it is good to change the tempo and style of a massage, and this is most true of percussive techniques, such as pummeling and cupping. With these invigorating movements, your aim is to stimulate the nerves and blood supply to the muscle, which may cause some redness. The techniques should not, however, be painful. Check with your partner as you work and beware of being too heavy-handed.

pummeling

❶ Make loose fists with your hands and place them on a large muscle such as the hamstrings.

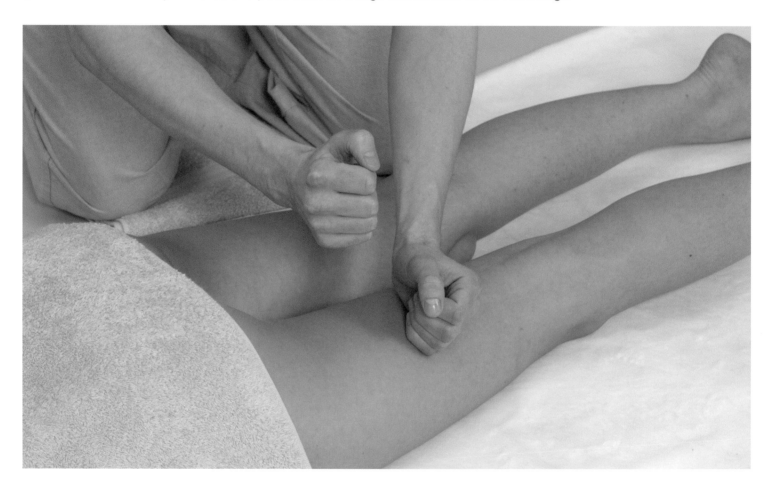

❷ Strike the muscle with alternate loose fists quite vigorously and quickly, building up a good rhythm and working over the whole area.

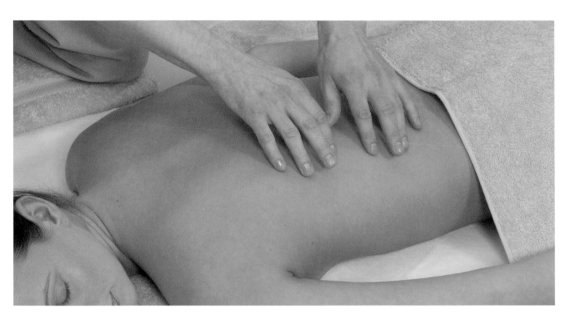

raindrops

Take an area of muscle and with both hands, using all ten fingers, quickly drum the fingertips all around the area, making the sound of falling rain. On delicate regions, such as the face, work lightly; to stimulate circulation in larger muscles, you can drum more firmly.

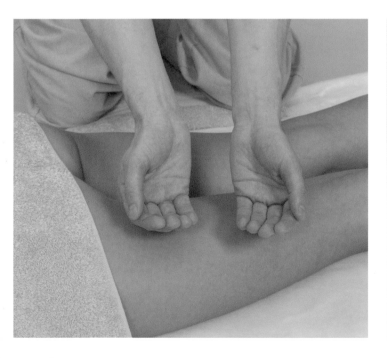

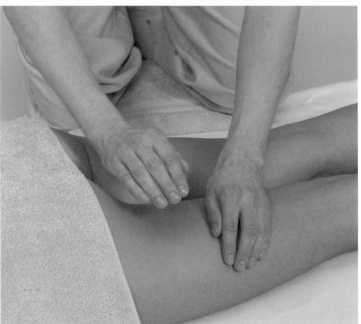

cupping

❶ Make cups with your hands by holding the fingers and thumbs of each hand together and curving the fingers up toward you.

❷ Place your cupped hands, facing down, on a large muscle and drum the body with alternate hands in a vigorous and stimulating fashion all over the muscle. The idea is to create a vacuum: the action of pulling away from the muscle stimulates the blood supply and nerves in the area.

cross-fiber fanning

One of the most effective ways to manipulate a muscle is to work across the muscle fibers. As you work, notice how the fibers of most muscles have a logical direction: the fibers of the arm and leg muscles, for instance, extend down the length of the limb. Armed with this knowledge, you can work safely on any muscle by massaging across the fibers.

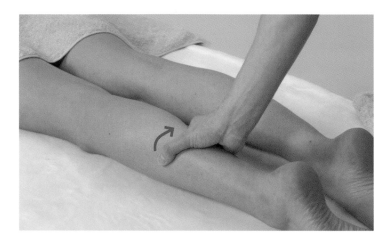

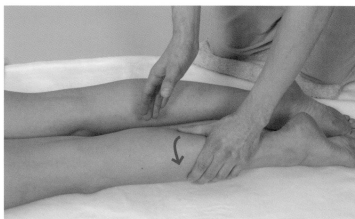

cross-fiber fanning with the thumb

Place the V of one hand flat on the muscle to be worked. Stretching the thumb away from the fingers and keeping the fingers still, roll the thumb across the muscle and fibers toward your fingers. Repeat with the other hand. Keeping constant contact, you can gradually work up the length of the muscle. On reaching the end of the muscle, glide the hands back down, ready to repeat.

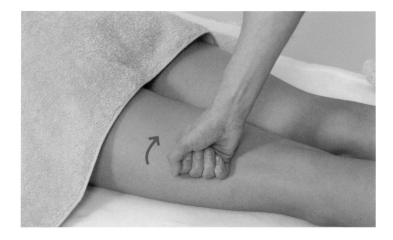

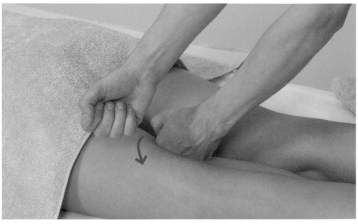

cross-fiber fanning with the fist

❶ To work on larger muscles, make fists with your hands. Place one hand on the muscle to be worked. Roll the back of one fist across the muscle and fibers.

❷ Repeat with the other fist in the opposite direction. Keeping your fists in constant contact with the skin, work gradually up the length of the muscle.

❸ When you reach the end of the muscle, glide both hands back down to the starting position, ready to repeat the stroke.

circling

Stroking the body is the best way to relax it, and we can apply this principle by performing large, slow, sweeping circles on the back and over limbs. When working on large areas, circle the hands, using a nice, even, rhythmic flow. To soothe and ease the body's joints and moisturize the skin with oil, use smaller fingertip circles.

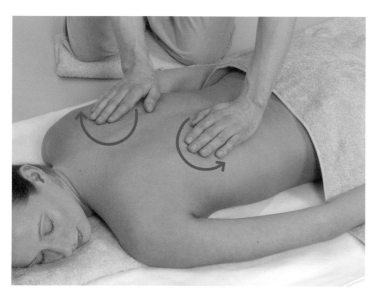

hand circles

Place both hands on the part of the body to be worked, fingers pointing away from you. Move your right hand upward and around to make a clockwise circle over the area. Circle the left hand counterclockwise.

fingertip circles

Circle your fingertips around the joints of the body—knees, elbows, wrists, ankles, hips, shoulders. There is no right or wrong way of doing this, so be creative and ask your partner for feedback on how good it feels.

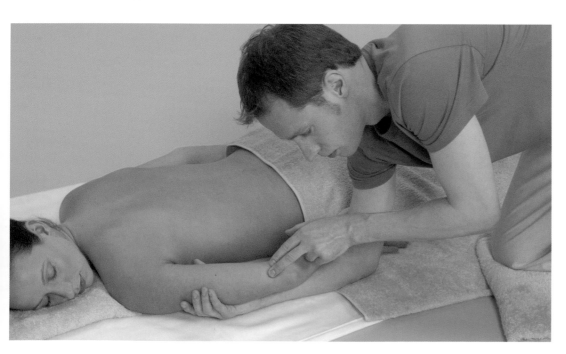

using the forearm

Massage does not have to rely solely on the use of your hands; the forearm is a very useful and powerful tool that can replace the hands when you want to give them a rest or manipulate muscles more deeply.

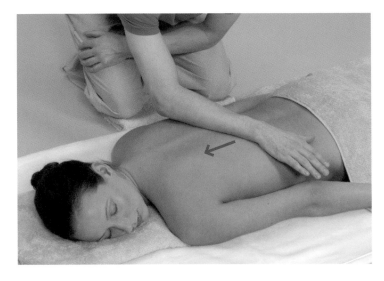

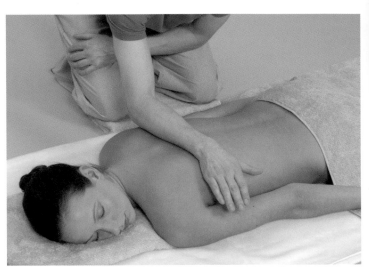

forearm effleurage
❶ Place your forearm on the muscle to be worked. Be careful with the spine.

❷ Leaning in with your body weight, sweep the forearm up the muscle with some pressure and gently back down to the starting position to repeat the stroke. Build up a sweeping motion similar to effleurage.

sawing
Using both arms, place the forearms on the muscle to be worked. Stroke forward and back, building up a sawing motion.

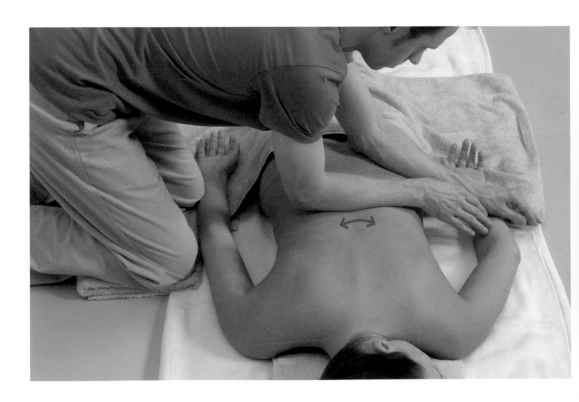

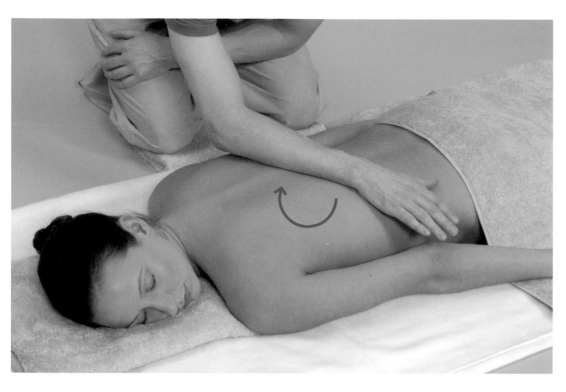

circling
Place your forearm on the muscle to be worked. Leaning in with your body weight, make a circular motion with your forearm all over the muscle.

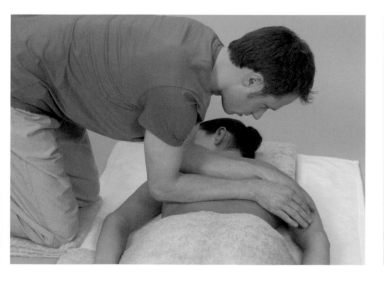

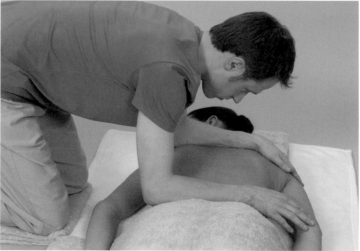

forearm stretch
❶ Rest both forearms side by side on the muscle to be worked. Lean in to the muscle, applying some body weight.

❷ Slowly glide both forearms away from each other to stretch the muscle. If the technique is performed rhythmically, you can lift both forearms off the body to reposition yourself, ready to start again.

cat paws, friction, and feathering

This compendium of techniques brings together strokes that are easy to learn and fun to perform. Use the cat paws technique, which takes its cue from a cat who has just landed in the lap and is preparing to settle down, to knead and pummel the muscles with the heels of the hands. If your massage partner is feeling cold to the touch, try some friction— a great way to warm the skin. Feathering guarantees to give your partner goose bumps in the nicest possible way.

cat paws

❶ Place the heels of both hands onto a large area of muscle and alternately push and pummel with each hand. It is possible to travel over a large area with this technique.

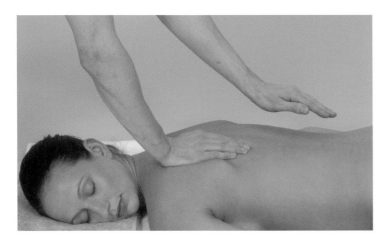

❷ Vary the pace, as performing this technique more quickly will be stimulating and useful to give at the end of a massage if someone needs to be active afterward.

friction rub

Place the blades of your hands together and rest them on the lower back. Very vigorously rub the muscle with the blades of the hands, moving each hand alternately in a brisk motion as if rubbing the hands together. Feel the heat begin to grow.

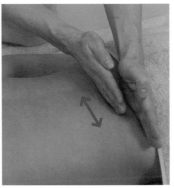 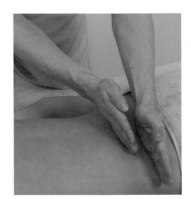

feathering

Place your fingertips very gently at the end of the muscle furthest away from you. Using featherweight strokes, feather the fingertips of one hand, then the other, over the skin, gradually working up the length of the muscle.

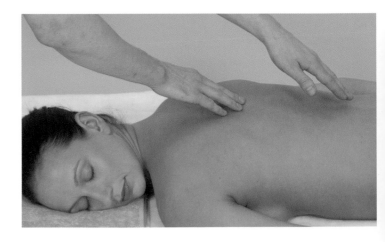

using the hands

You now know some of the essential massage techniques used in this book. In the massage programs that follow in Parts 3, 4, and 5, I refer frequently to various parts of the hands commonly used in massage, but not in everyday life. Here is a visual guide to identifying those different areas.

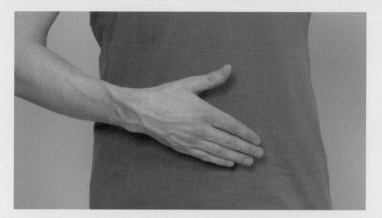

The V of the hand
The web of skin found between the index finger and thumb

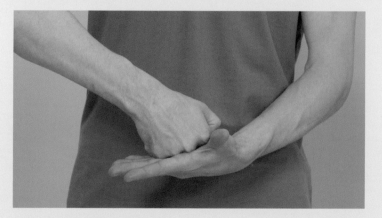

The flat of the knuckle
The part of the fist created by the first bones of the fingers

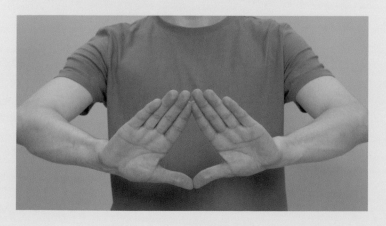

The triangle
A triangle created by placing the two thumbs and two index fingers together

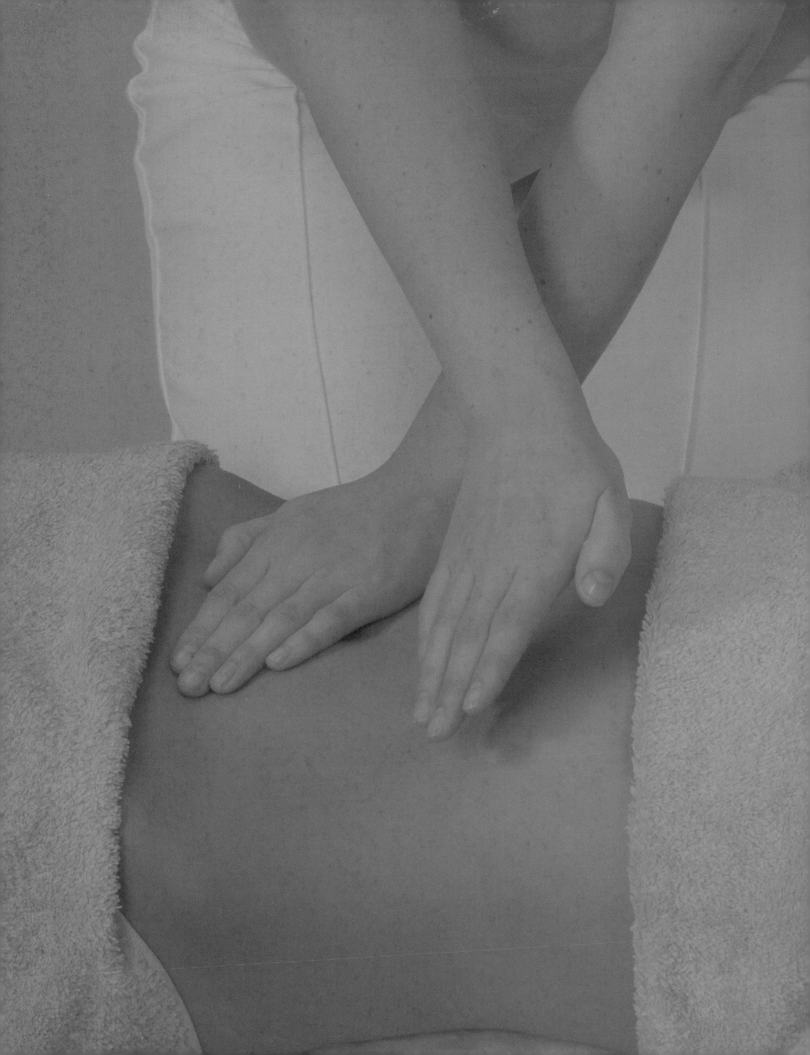

body-specific massage

Once you have familiarized yourself with the techniques in Part 2, you may want to add in some additional techniques to your repertoire for variety.

the back

Many of us hold much of our tension in the back and it therefore makes sense to begin a massage here. Sitting or standing still for long periods throughout the day can cause the muscles of the back to tighten; massage helps relieve this and is deeply relaxing for the whole body, mind, and spirit. If you only have half an hour or so to spare for massage, a back massage is extremely effective. Working on the erector spinae muscles on either side of the spine stimulates nerves that radiate out to the rest of the body, revitalizing and rebalancing every part of the body.

CAUTION: Never apply any pressure to the spine itself.

starting position: Ask your partner to lie comfortably on his or her front, and cover the back and legs with towels, tucking them into your partner's underwear for warmth.

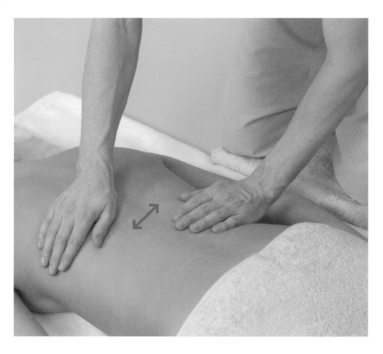

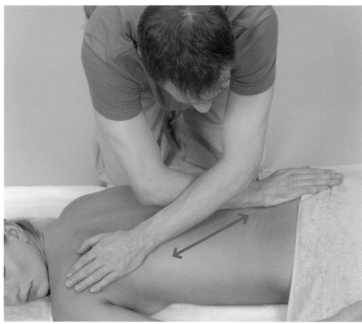

scrub (no oil)

To warm the body and prepare it for massage, start with a vigorous, warming scrub.

❶ Position yourself by your companion's side, and place both hands on the back, perpendicular to the body.

❷ With quick, vigorous movements, rub the hands across the width of the back, traveling up and down the length of it.

diagonal stretch

Many of us are shorter in the evening than when we got out of bed in the morning. Over the course of the day, the disks between the vertebrae compress and fluid drains from them. Once you have warmed the body with the scrub technique, stretch the muscles of the back in order to lengthen them.

❶ Still kneeling by your partner's side, cross your arms and place one hand onto the shoulder blade, the other onto the opposite buttock.

❷ Lean over your partner and use your body weight to stretch outward slowly; hold for a few seconds. Release slowly, then repeat on the other side.

effleurage for the back

Fold the towels back and coat the back with oil, using gentle, even strokes. Ensure you get a nice sheen all over, including on the sides, neck, beneath the shoulders, and on the buttocks. Many people hold tension in the buttocks, particularly if they have a lower-back problem or do a lot of exercise. However, some people may not feel comfortable having the gluteal muscles of the buttocks massaged, so respect their modesty.

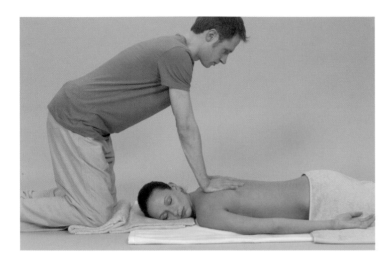

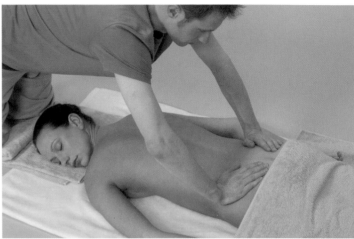

❶ Position yourself by the crown of your partner's head. Place both hands on the upper back on either side of the spine, fingers and thumbs together and pointing toward the buttocks. Ensure your thumbs are approximately 1½ inches apart from each other.

❸ When you reach the top of the buttocks, sweep your hands outward toward the hips, ready to glide up the sides of your partner's back. If your partner prefers that you do not work on the buttocks, you can finish the stroke earlier, at the curve of the lower back.

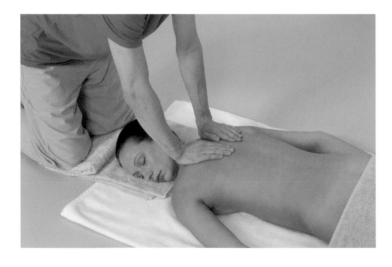

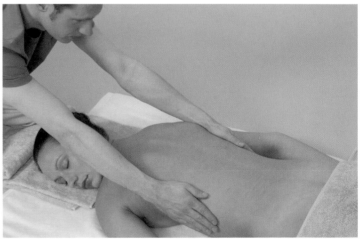

❷ Glide your hands firmly down the back on either side of the spine at a slow, even pace. Lean in with your body weight, keeping the pressure firmly applied through the whole palm.

❹ Bring your hands up the outer sides of the back, leaning backward and using your body weight to assist you. Keep a nice, slow pace as you glide your hands toward your partner's shoulder joints.

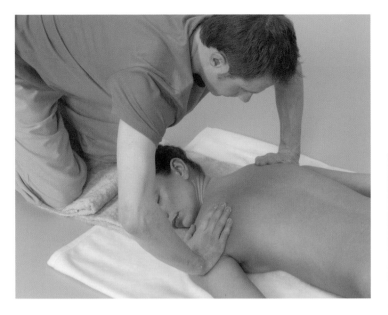

❺ Lighten the pressure upon reaching the shoulders, rotating your hands so that your wrists and elbows point outward. Cupping your hands around the contours of the body, stroke your hands down the top of the arms over the deltoid muscles that cap the shoulder joints.

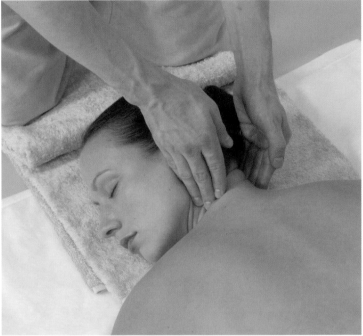

❼ Glide firmly up the sides of the neck, still with strong fingers, avoiding the cervical spine in the back of the neck, and the throat. Take your fingertips all the way up to the base of the skull (usually indicated by the hairline), ensuring that your partner does not mind getting oil in the hair.

❽ You are now ready to repeat the stroke. Glide your hands gently down the neck and flow straight into the next stroke. Repeat from step 1, breathing out on the downward stroke and in on the return stroke to help relax both you and your partner.

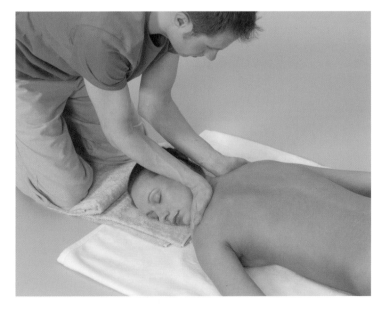

❻ Turn your hands 180 degrees so your wrists lead your fingers back up the arm. Allow the fingers to scoop beneath the shoulders. At this point, tense your fingers so they are strong and rigid and scoop deeply into the trapezius muscles. This area can hold a lot of tension and your partner will appreciate deeper pressure now to help release tightness.

open-handed kneading on the neck

In this technique, you really dance with your partner, so adopt the half-kneeling position (page 22), which allows you to maximize the effectiveness of your body movements. Make sure to apply pressure evenly throughout the V of the hand as you work.

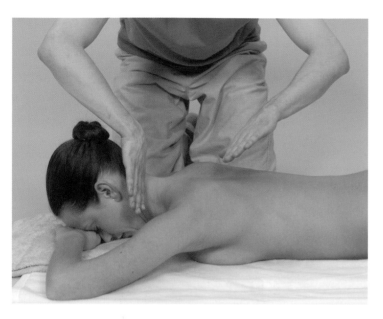

❶ Position yourself facing your partner's right side by the neck. In order to expose your partner's neck fully, you may need to ask him or her to place both hands, palms down, beneath the forehead.

❷ Hold the fingers of your right hand together and stretch your thumb away from them to form a V. Use the V to scoop into the muscles of the back of the neck close to the head. Continue to scoop down the length of the neck, applying firm pressure with the web of the hand.

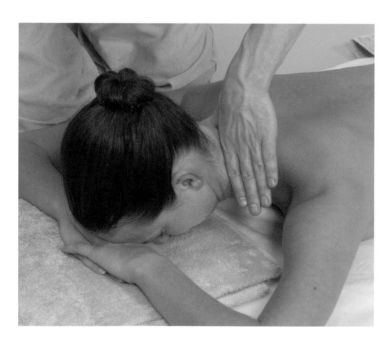

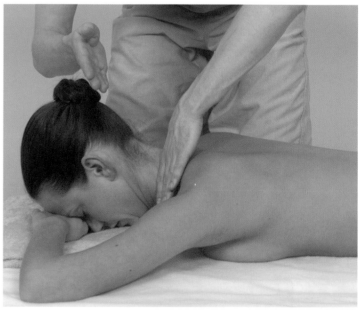

❸ As the right hand finishes the stroke, make a V with your left hand and repeat the stroke in the opposite direction, scooping up the neck muscle and into the hairline.

❹ Repeat the movement. As one hand finishes the action, let the other take over. Allow your body to rock from side to side as your hands move in one direction and then the other.

alternate kneading on the upper back

Shoulders can be the number one area for tension, so it is invaluable to spend time easing muscles here. Sometimes the most effective thing to do is work the muscle for a while, leave it to focus on another part of the body, then come back to it. Relaxation is most likely to occur in the rest period.

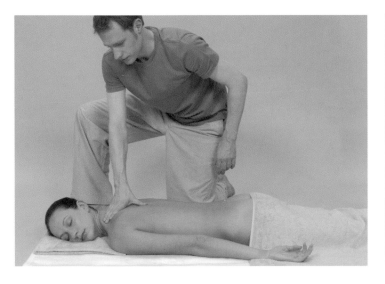

❶ Kneeling by your partner's side, glide one hand over the upper back on the side of the spine opposite you.

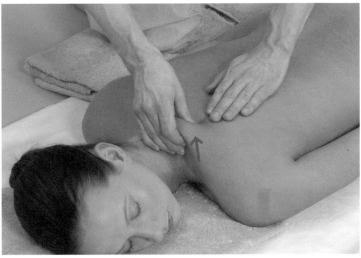

❸ When you can no longer pull the muscle, allow it to slip from your grasp and glide your fingers over the upper back toward you. As that hand continues toward you, move in with the other hand to take over the massage.

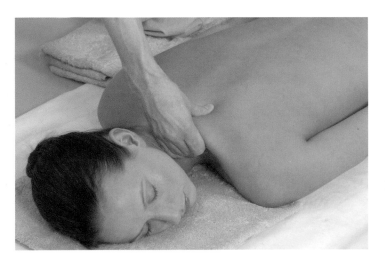

❷ Grab the trapezius muscle between your fingers and thumb, and pull toward you, anchoring your thumb on the muscle of the upper back. This feels tight for most people, so ask for feedback. Remember you're aiming at pleasurable pain.

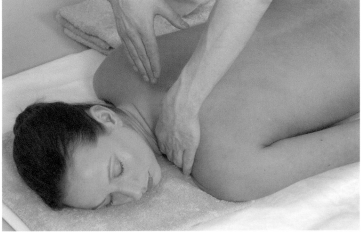

❹ Repeat the technique with the other hand, allowing your hands to get into a rhythm of alternately gliding and pulling. Once you have finished on this side, move around to the other side of the body and repeat on that side.

thai seat

It is important to be comfortable when giving a massage, so make yourself at home and turn your companion's feet into a seat. You'll be surprised to hear that most people feel quite comfortable with this, and it's an easy position from which to apply static pressure using your body weight.

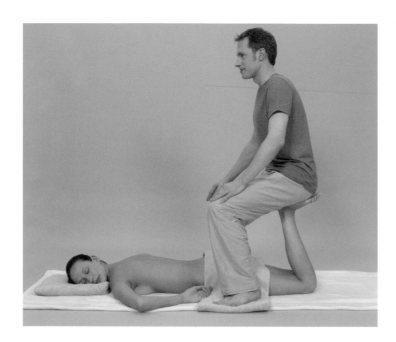

❶ Bend your partner's legs at the knee and sit on the soles of the feet. Ensure this is comfortable for your companion.

❷ Place one thumb on either side of the spine and lean in with some body pressure. Hold the pressure for a few seconds, then gently release.

❸ Repeat the technique all the way up the back, then glide your hands back down to the starting position to repeat.

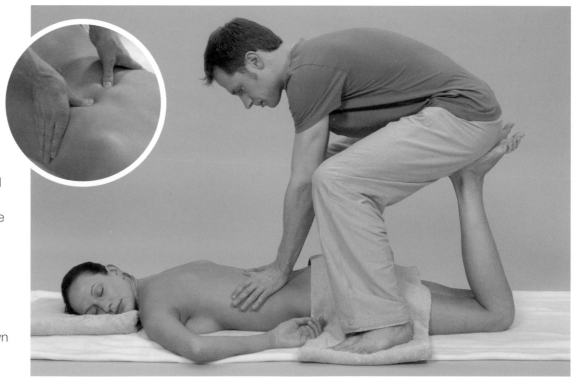

sawing the shoulder blades

Several muscles attach to the shoulder blades. Massage is beneficial here, as the muscles can get very tight, particularly for those who sit working at a desk for long periods.

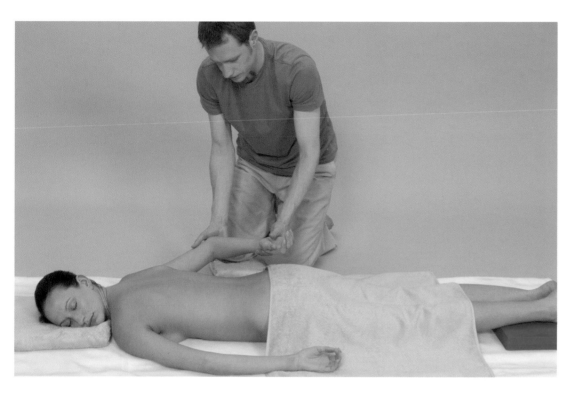

❶ Position yourself by your partner's side. To make the shoulder blades stick out like an angel's wing, very carefully take your partner's arm and rest it on the lower back. Be sure to support at the elbow and take the entire weight of the arm; your partner should not have to do anything.

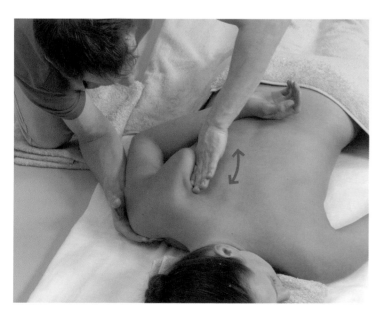

❷ With the V of your hand, which fits nicely around the shoulder blade, carve into the muscle with the web of the hand, using a sawing motion forward and back. Repeat on the other arm.

❸ Follow with the rolling pressure on pages 44–45, working all around this area.

circular pressure

The lower back is a vulnerable place for many people and a common site of injury and weakness. You can place a cushion beneath the abdomen to offer support to a weak back before performing the next technique, which uses the heel of the hand.

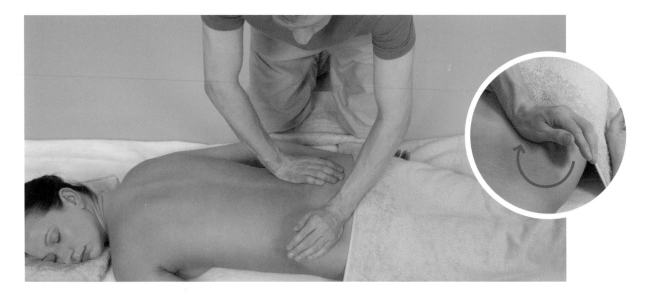

❶ Still positioned by your partner's side, rest your nonworking hand close to the muscle about to be worked. Slightly cock your other hand at the wrist and lean in with your body weight to apply pressure to the gluteals with the heel of your hand.

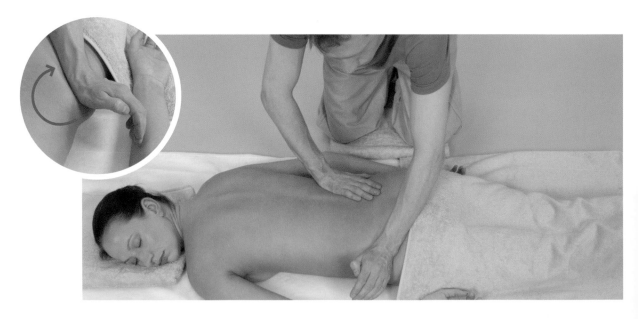

❷ Perform a circling motion that initiates from your shoulder, making three or four spiraling circles over the muscle, gradually working outward. When you reach the outside of the muscle, lift the hand off, ready to repeat again.

spiraling pressure

Some people find the gluteal area very tender, so ask for lots of feedback about pressure from your partner. This technique can be applied all over the buttocks area with your partner's agreement.

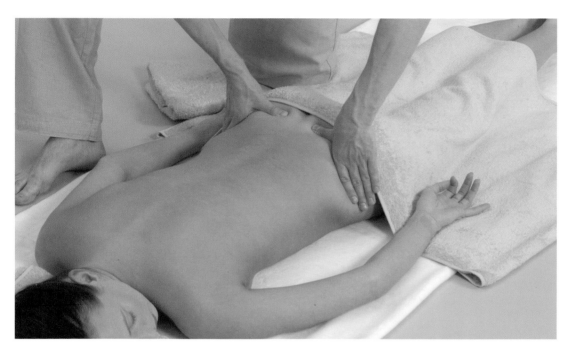

❶ Position yourself by your partner's gluteal muscles at the buttocks, facing up the body. Place each thumb at the top of each buttock on either side of the spine. Keep your fingers relaxed, resting on the side of the buttocks.

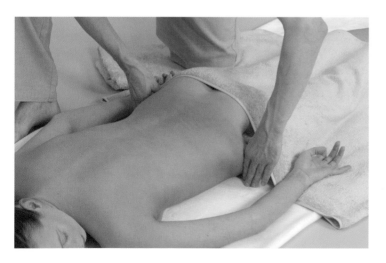

❷ Leaning in with your body weight, apply pressure with your thumbs so that they sink deeply into the muscle to a level that your partner can tolerate. Make between four and six deep, slow, spiral movements into these gluteal muscles, gradually working outward toward the hips. The right thumb circles clockwise, the left counterclockwise, with the most pressure at the top of the circle.

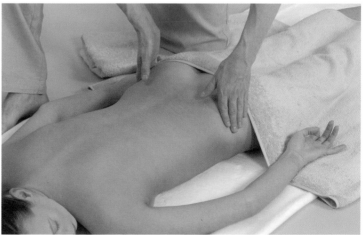

❸ When you reach the outside of the buttocks, lift your thumbs and glide your hands back in toward the center. Repeat the action, moving from the center of the buttocks out toward the hips. Try to lean your body weight over your thumbs on the initial part of the movement so that you do not rely purely on the strength of your thumbs.

alternate kneading on the buttocks

Here you knead the muscles of the buttock furthest away from you with a kneading movement similar to that used on the upper back (page 65).

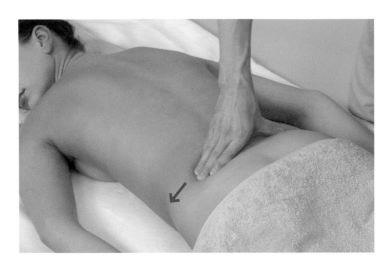

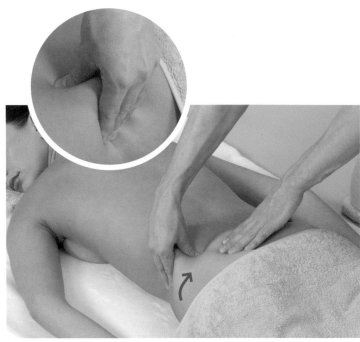

❶ Position yourself alongside your partner, facing the buttocks. Place one hand on the center of the buttock furthest away from you and push the muscle of the buttock away from the bone toward the hip.

❷ Trap the muscle between your fingers and thumb. Keep the thumb still, and using your fingers, pull the muscle back toward the thumb. The thumb acts as an anchor to pull the muscle against, remaining stationary as far as possible. Taking care not to pinch, gradually let the bulk of the muscle "slip" from your fingers.

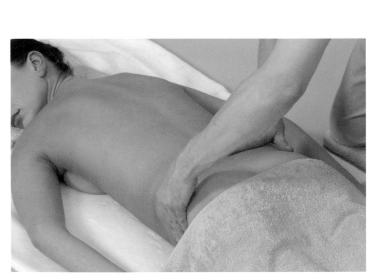

❸ Glide your hand toward you and repeat the movement with the other hand on the same buttock. As one hand leaves, the other takes over.

❹ Continue the technique, alternating hands. Rock forward as you push the muscle away from you, and backward as you draw the flesh back over your thumb. Keep the rhythm smooth, one hand following the other. Once you have finished, move around to the other side of the body to repeat on the other side.

open-handed kneading on the lower back

This technique feels really comforting on an aching lower back. It is very similar to the technique performed on the neck on page 62.

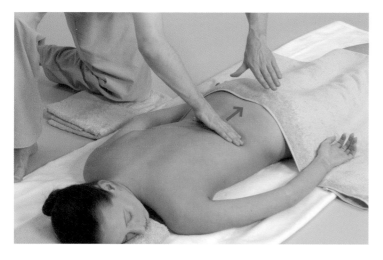

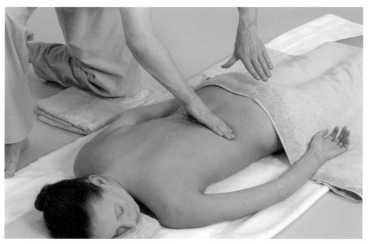

① Adopt the half-kneeling position (page 22) by your partner's lower back and facing the body. Place the V of one hand over the hollowing curve of the lower back.

② Scoop into the lower back with the V of your hand, leaning in with your body weight.

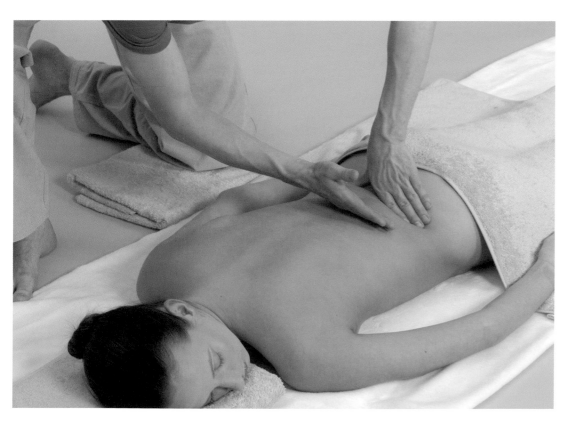

③ As the first hand finishes the stroke, repeat the movement with your other hand, but scooping in the opposite direction. Work rocking or swaying with the technique to enhance its effectiveness and to make the stroke relaxing for both giver and recipient.

pulling up

Once all the muscles in the back have been loosened up, it feels wonderful to have them lifted away from the bones. This is a very simple, yet satisfying technique to perform.

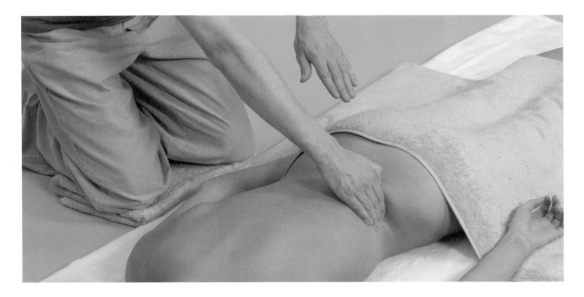

❶ Position yourself by the center of your partner's back, facing the body. Start at the gluteal muscles of the buttocks if your partner is in agreement. Place one hand on the gluteal muscle and pull firmly and slowly. As this first hand finishes the movement, repeat the action with your other hand.

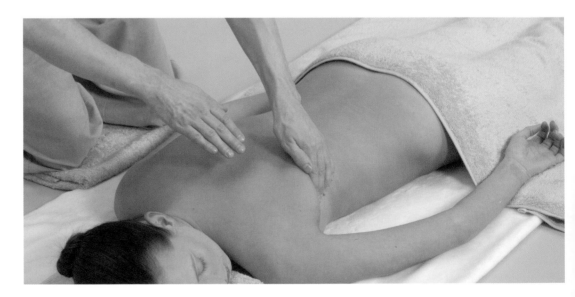

❷ Take the technique all the way up the length of the side of the back and onto the shoulder, then move back down the body. Once you have made several repetitions, move around the body to perform the action on the other side.

one thousand hands

This is a variation of the effleurage movement, using the flat of both hands with fingers and thumbs touching. It is called "one thousand hands" because that is exactly how it should feel to the recipient. Perform the movement very slowly as a conclusion to your back-massage sequence.

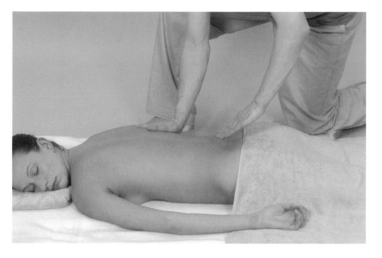

❶ Position yourself at your partner's side, level with the hips and facing the head. Glide your right hand up the right side of your partner's back, about 1½ inches away from the spine. Continue up toward the shoulder.

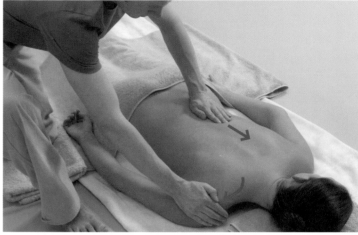

❷ As you approach the shoulder, glide your hands up and outward over the top of the shoulder. When the hand comes around the top of the right arm, place your left hand on the left side of the lower back.

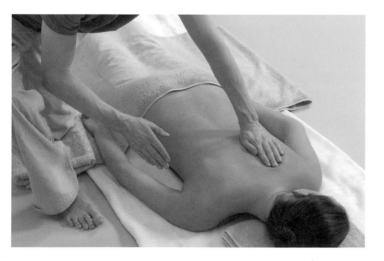

❸ Begin to glide your left hand up the left side of the back and gently lift the right hand away. Repeat the stroke, one hand moving upward on your partner's back at all times, so it feels like one continuous stroke. Position yourself as you work so you can cover the whole back, rocking forward with each of the up strokes.

other techniques for the back

- All pressure on any tight muscles (page 45–47)
- Rolling pressure on the rhomboid shoulder-blade muscles (page 47)
- Wringing across the width of the back (page 48)
- Combing (page 49)
- Raking (page 49)
- Pummeling on the gluteal muscles (page 50)
- Cupping on the gluteal muscles of the buttocks (page 51)
- Circling (page 53)
- Forearm stroking (page 54)
- Forearm stretch (page 55)
- Friction rub, particularly good on the curve of the lower back (page 56)
- Cat paws (page 56)
- Feathering (page 56)

the legs

The legs work so hard in standing and walking, it comes as no surprise to learn that they benefit enormously from massage. The blood supply has a long way to travel back up the leg toward the heart, and deep, sweeping effleurage is incredibly beneficial in assisting this return. When massaging the leg, work with the limb in two parts, focusing on the calf and thigh separately. Perform all the techniques in Part 2 on the calf first and then the thigh.

CAUTION: Never apply pressure or manipulation on or below a varicose vein.

back of the leg

starting position: Ask your partner to lie on his or her front, and cover well with towels to maintain body temperature. Fold back the towel to expose the leg nearest you. With even strokes, apply oil to the leg, looking for varicose veins on the upper and lower leg.

effleurage for the back of the leg

Ask your partner for feedback as you increase the pressure on each repetition of this stroke.

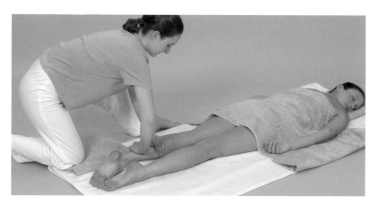

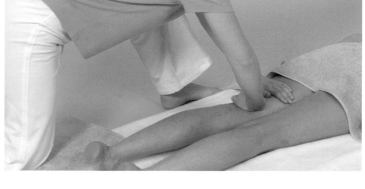

❶ Kneel next to your partner's ankles, facing the head. With fingers pointing in, cup your hands, one above the other, around the calf with the outside hand leading. The outside hand is the hand that will stroke around the outside of the leg and leads because it has farther to travel than the inside hand.

❸ When you reach the top of the leg, fan your hands out to each side of the leg and pull gently back down to the ankle.

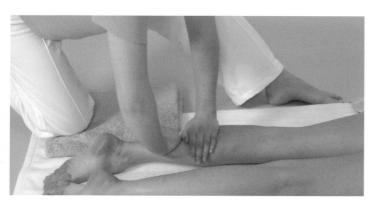

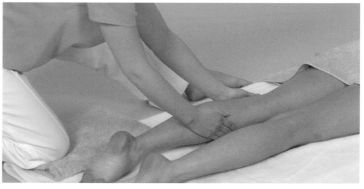

❷ Glide your hands firmly and slowly up the calf. Release the pressure over the back of the knee and continue firmly up toward the buttock.

❹ It really helps to lean into the technique as you work up the leg and to lean backward as your hands return to the ankle. Repeat, increasing pressure a little on each subsequent repetition.

fist stroking

This technique helps to relax the hamstring muscles at the back of the thigh, which, if they are tense, can adversely affect posture.

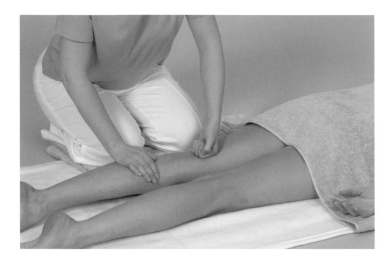

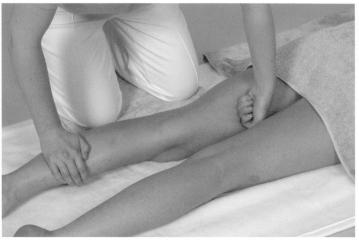

❶ Still positioned next to your partner's leg, lightly rest the hand nearest your partner on the calf. With your other hand, create a fist. Place the fist on the lower thigh, ready to massage with the flat of your knuckles. Adjust your positioning to allow your body weight to increase your pressure into the muscle.

❸ Move your fist to the inside of the thigh, repeating the stroke slowly and deeply from above the knee to the top of the thigh. Repeat the action several times.

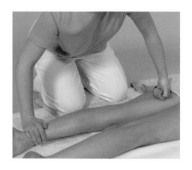 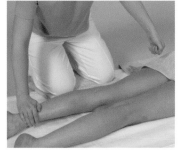

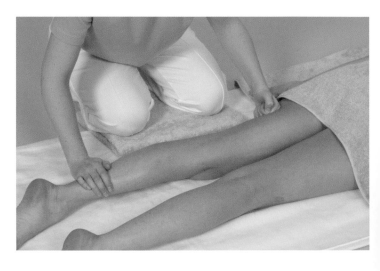

❷ Lean into the muscle, stroking firmly and slowly up the back of the thigh from above the knee all the way into the gluteal muscles of the buttock. Maintaining contact with your resting hand on the calf, lift your fist away from the thigh. Repeat the movement several times in a rhythmic fashion up the center of the thigh.

❹ Repeat the stroke on the outer thigh. Take care not to apply pressure to the hip joint as you work here.

muscle rolling

Wearing high-heeled shoes can cause the muscles of the calves to shorten, often making them feel tight. This technique helps ease out tension in the calves and is especially effective if performed after exercise to help prevent stiffness in the muscles of the thighs and calves. Your partner may find this painful, so ask for lots of feedback.

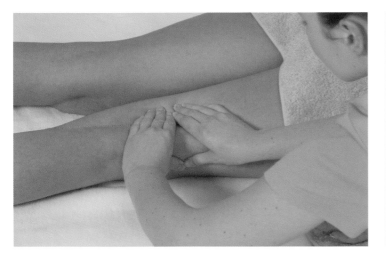

❶ Face your partner's thigh and imagine a nine-box grid on the back of the thigh. Form a triangle with your thumbs and index fingers and place your hands, palms down, on the thigh in the left-hand corner of the grid.

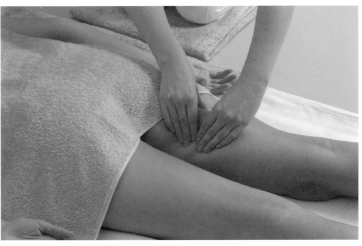

❸ Without moving your fingers, stretch your thumbs away again to re-create the triangle and repeat the rolling action several times. Move the triangle to each square in turn and repeat the technique until you have covered the whole thigh.

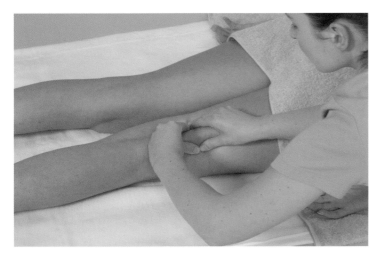

❷ Press down and grasp some muscle. Ensure that you are grabbing muscle and not just skin to avoid pinching. While keeping your fingers still, slide your thumbs toward your fingers, "rolling" the muscle until your thumb and fingers meet.

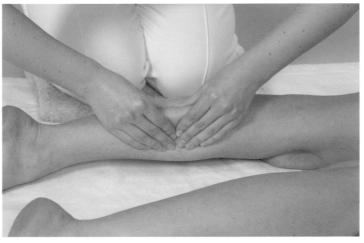

❹ If desired, repeat the technique on the gastrocnemius muscle in the calf.

transverse pressure up the calf

As you work on this technique, constantly ask your partner for feedback and proceed with care, as some people find the action very painful. At no time should you apply pressure to the back of the knee.

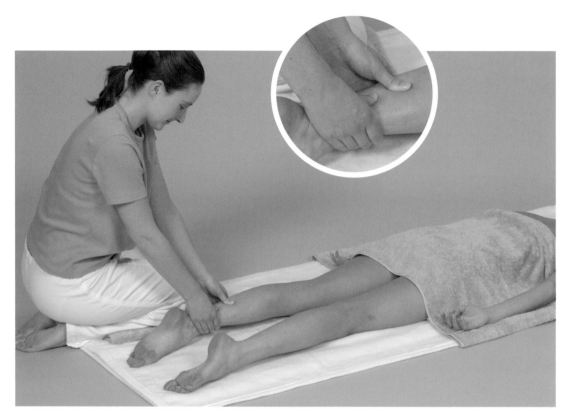

❶ Kneel beside the calf and face your partner's head. Place one thumb on the calf, just above your partner's ankle on the center of the gastrocnemius muscle. Keep your fingers relaxed, resting on the side of the leg.

❷ Glide your thumb slowly and firmly up the calf to just below the knee. Your fingers should slide gently up the sides of the leg as the thumbs move up the calf.

❸ Before you reach the back of the knee, gently glide your hand back down the calf, ready to repeat the technique. Build up a slow but regular rhythm, leaning forward as you move up the calf and leaning backward as the hand returns toward the ankle.

❹ If desired, repeat the stroke all over the back of the calf. Then soothe the calf with effleurage strokes as before (page 75).

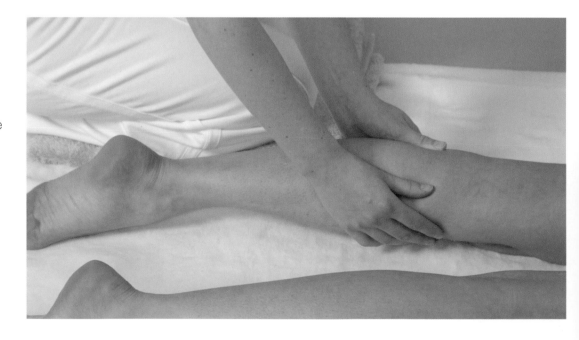

scoops

As the gastrocnemius muscle of the calf is a long muscle that can have concentrated areas of tension, it is effective to scoop into the muscle and compress it against the underlying bone, thereby squeezing out the tension. Lactic acid that can build up in the muscle will also be released from the fibers and flushed from the body.

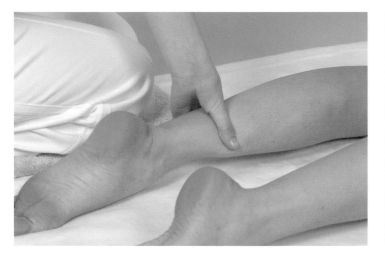

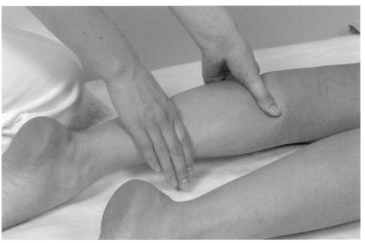

❶ Still positioned beside your partner's leg, place the V of your hand on the lower calf. Sweep it all the way to the top of the thigh, taking care not to exert any pressure over the back of the knee.

❷ As the first hand is about to leave the top of the thigh, repeat the movement with the other hand, sweeping up from the lower calf to the top of the thigh and maintaining contact with one hand throughout the movement.

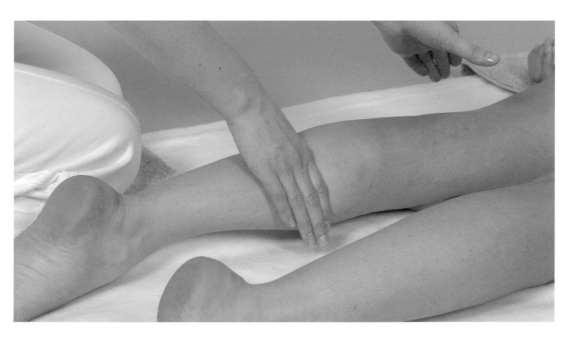

❸ Alternatively, apply this technique in the same way, but using very small sweeps from the lower calf to the top of the thigh, and working more briskly.

working with a bent leg

By bending the leg at the knee, the calf muscles become very relaxed and easier to manipulate. As well as the techniques here, experiment with strokes from Part 2 from this position: try the pressure techniques, raking with one hand, and circling. Sometimes, when other techniques have not succeeded in loosening a stiff muscle, it is useful to go back to the simplest of methods, such as a static hold. The lack of movement in this hold can be deeply relaxing, especially for those who don't have much stillness in everyday life.

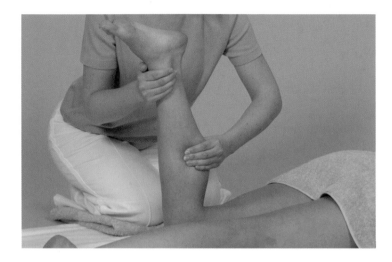

static holds
❶ Positioned next to your partner's leg, bend the knee and support the calf by holding the ankle. Ensure the calf is at a right angle to the floor.

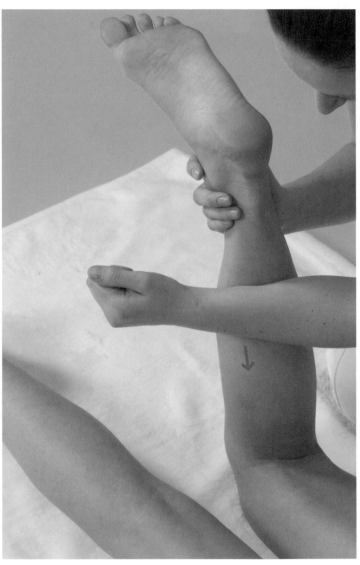

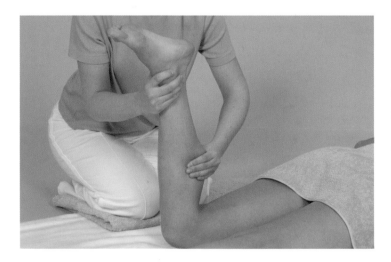

❷ With your other hand, pinch into the muscles of the calf, starting close to the knee. Hold the muscles for a few seconds and slowly release. Repeat, working down toward the ankle and holding in a number of places.

forearm pressure
Keeping the leg bent, apply pressure with your forearm, starting at the ankle and working down the calf toward the knee. When your arm reaches just below the knee, lift it away and take it back to the ankle to repeat the stroke.

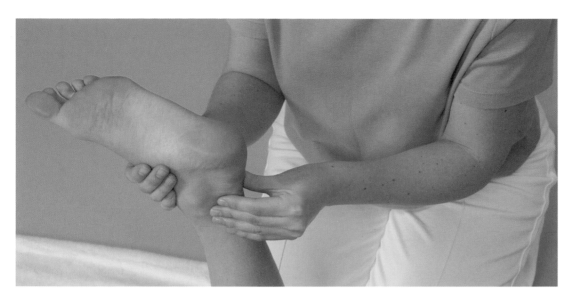

kneading the Achilles tendon

With fingertips and thumb, manipulate the Achilles tendon by pressing in and pulling away, using a small circular motion. This helps to loosen a very taut tendon, which is prone to snapping in sports injuries.

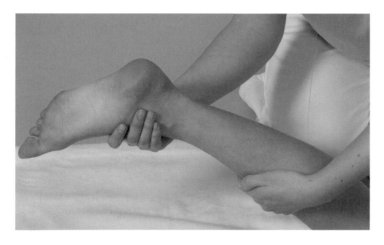

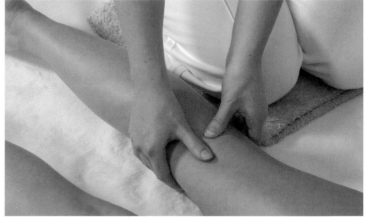

circling the back of the knee

❶ Take the leg slowly back down to the floor, supporting the full weight of the limb for your relaxed partner.

❷ Sandwich the sides of the knee with the fingers of both hands and apply gentle, circular pressure with both thumbs into the back of the knee. Take great care, and be wary of applying too much pressure to this vulnerable and much-neglected area.

finishing touches

End work on this leg with more effleurage strokes (page 75), then repeat all the techniques from page 75 onward on the other leg.

front of the leg

starting position: Carefully help your partner onto his or her back and replace the towels. Position yourself beside your partner's leg, facing toward the head, and uncover the leg nearest you. Evenly apply oil to the leg.

effleurage for the front of the leg

As before, start your work on this part of the leg with long, soothing strokes.

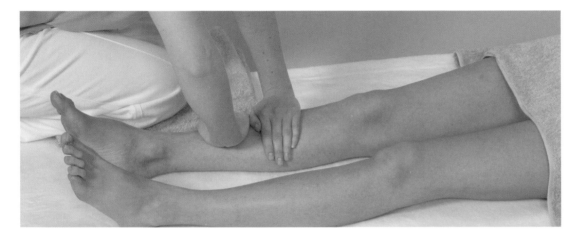

❶ Follow the effleurage technique on page 75 to work on the front of the leg, but apply less pressure on the calf and glide carefully over the knee.

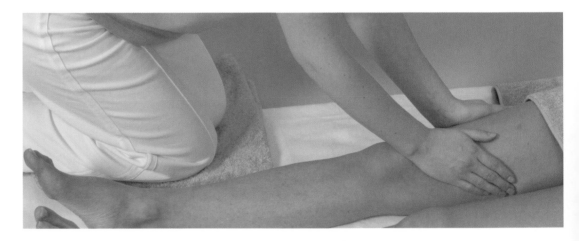

❷ Keeping the pace of the stroke slow but regular and with even pressure, repeat it rhythmically to relax your partner. Breathe out on the upward stroke and in on the return stroke to further relax both you and your partner.

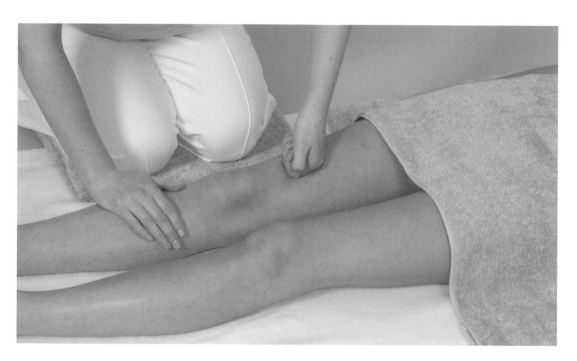

fist stroking the thigh

Follow the technique on page 76, continuing to work only above the knee on the quadriceps muscles. As these muscles can be very tight, ask for feedback before you work too deeply into the muscles and remember to respect your partner's modesty when stroking up the inner thigh.

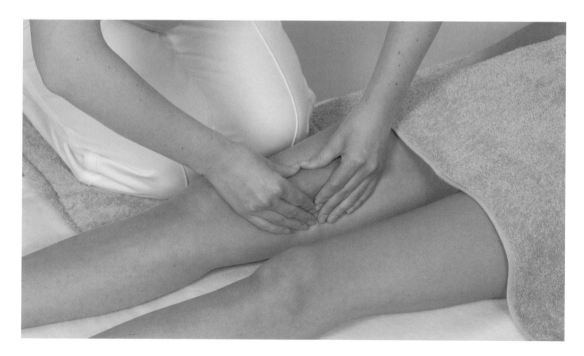

muscle rolling

Follow the technique on page 77, using the nine-box grid in exactly the same way.

massaging the knee

These techniques soothe and relax the knees, but be wary of applying too much pressure on the patella, or kneecap, itself, and do not perform the techniques on people with a history of dislocation of the knee.

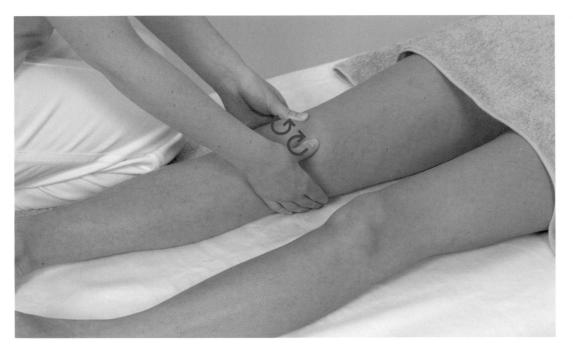

work around the knee
Position yourself beside your partner's knees. Place your hands on the leg so that your thumbs lie below the patella. Lightly stroke your thumbs over the patella and sweep around the outside of the bone and back to your starting position.

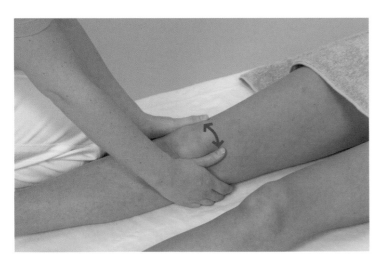

nudging the patella
Sandwich the knee by placing your hands on either side of the leg. With your thumbs sitting one on each side of the patella, nudge the bone from side to side very gently to encourage mobility. If there is little or no movement, do not force it.

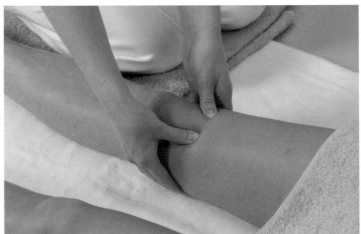

pressure
Keeping your fingers in the same position as for the last technique, circle the thumbs with pressure into the muscles above and surrounding the knee. Because you are working on tendons, this area may feel taut.

circular pressure

The large calf muscle known as the gastrocnemius is attached to the bones of the calf. Applying circular pressure with the heel of the hand stretches the muscle away from the bone to aid relaxation and lengthening of the muscle.

❶ Positioned beside your partner's lower leg, support the outside of the calf with one hand and place the heel of the other hand on the gastrocnemius muscle, close to the ankle.

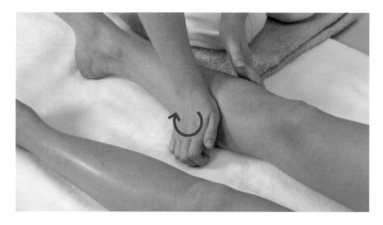 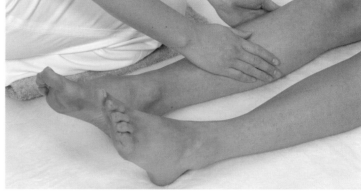

❷ With a small, circular motion, work into the muscle with the heel of your hand. Make a spiraling movement that allows you to travel up the calf to just below the knee.

❸ Gently stroke down with a flat hand to soothe the leg and return to your starting position, ready to repeat the stroke.

finishing touches

End the massage for the front of the legs as you started, using effleurage (page 82). Then perform all the techniques from page 75 onward on the other leg.

other techniques for the legs

- All pressure techniques on tight muscles (page 78)
- Wringing across the width of the thigh on the front and back of the legs, and on the back of the calves (page 48)
- Pummeling on the front and back of the thighs (page 50)
- Cupping on the front and back of the thighs (page 51)
- Raindrops all over the legs (page 51)
- Cross-fiber fanning on the front and back of the thighs and the back of the calves (page 52)
- Forearm stroking on the front and back of the thighs (page 54)
- Forearm stretch along the length of the back of the legs (page 55)
- Cat paws all over the back of the leg, gliding over the knees (page 56)
- Feathering all over the legs (page 56)

the feet

You may find it surprising to learn that we compress twenty-six bones into each shoe every day. Massaging out the tension this creates can be incredibly relaxing—it has to be my favorite form of the therapy. Having someone pay his or her undivided attention to such a small area of the body is divine! Because there are so many bones in the foot, we spend some time in this sequence gently manipulating and easing out the joints between all those tiny bones. When performing a foot massage, remember to apply firm pressure to avoid tickling your partner. Perform all the techniques on one foot, then shift position, if necessary, to work on the other foot.

starting position: Ask your partner to lie on his or her back. If necessary, place a pillow or rolled-up towel beneath the knees for extra comfort and support for the lower back. Cover the entire body with towels to retain warmth. Kneel facing the soles of the feet and uncover one foot, keeping the rest of the leg well covered. Apply a tiny amount of oil to the foot using firm, even strokes. Too much oil will make the stretches we do on the foot less effective.

effleurage for the feet

Keep your strokes firm, building up to a reassuring rhythm as you glide, fan out, sweep, and circle.

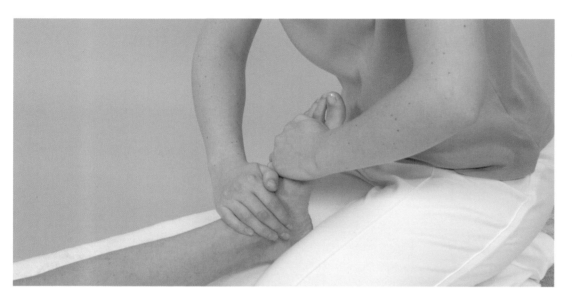

❶ Place your hands one above the other over the toes, fingers pointing in toward the center. Glide your hands up toward the ankle.

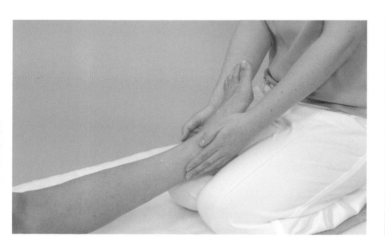

❷ Fan both hands out, sweeping around the ankle joint, then circle around the joint with your fingertips several times.

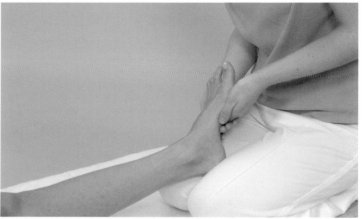

❸ Cup your hands underneath the foot with little fingers touching, and sweep your hands along the sole of the foot from heel to toes.

ankle rotation

To make this movement effective, it is important to keep the whole of your hand in contact with the arch of the foot, so make sure to establish a firm hold before you start to rotate.

❶ With one hand, take hold of the foot by grasping the arch of the foot between the fingers and thumb of one hand. Support beneath the ankle by cupping the heel with your other hand.

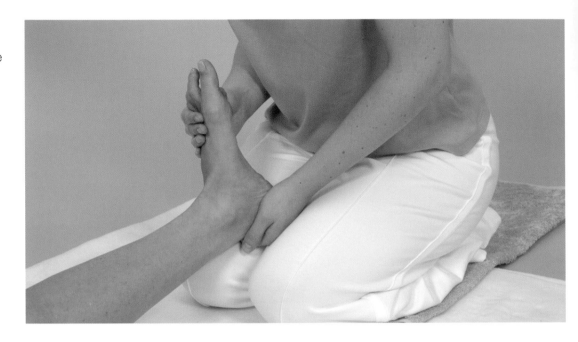

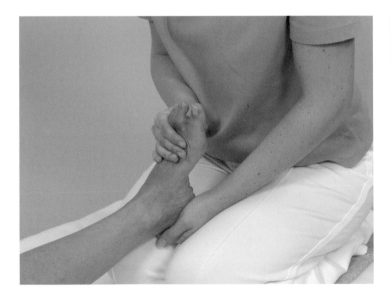

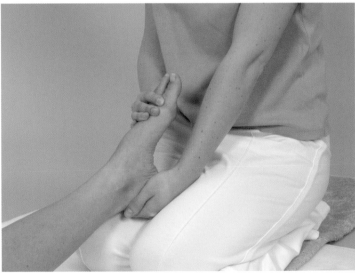

❷ Rotate the foot from the ankle slowly by using the circling motion of your own body to encourage the circling of your upper hand. This feels strange, as if you are working against a great deal of resistance. Asking for feedback from your partner, gently increase the arc of the circle as far as the foot will allow, keeping the pace slow but constant.

❸ Make five or six circles in one direction. Repeat the action, rotating the foot in the opposite direction, again moving slowly and gently, and aiming to increase the arc of the circle of rotation.

corkscrew

This movement takes its name from the action it mimics—that of turning a corkscrew. Most feet can take a lot of pressure, but ask your partner for feedback while you work, as it is possible to hit a sore spot.

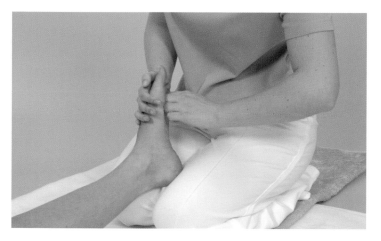

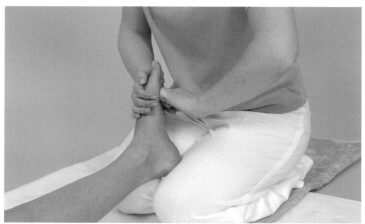

❶ Cupping the top of the foot with one hand, make a fist with the other hand. Use the sharp edge of your knuckles to press into the sole, supporting the foot with your cupped hand.

❷ Make the action of one turn of a corkscrew with your fist, moving as far as your wrist will allow.

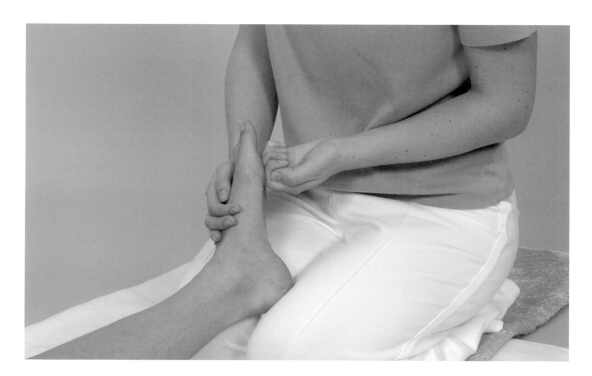

❸ Once you have fully turned your wrist, release the pressure and move your hand up the sole a little. Repeat the corkscrew technique slowly all over the sole. Use the hand cupping the top of the foot as a support to push against.

fist stroking

Continuing to support the top of the foot with one hand, again make a fist with the other hand.

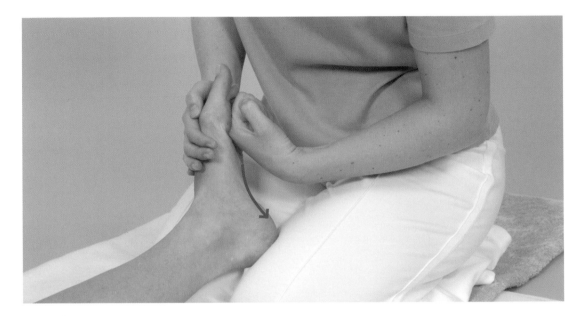

❶ Place your fist on the top of the sole so that the inside of the wrist faces you. Slowly stroke down the sole of the foot, from underneath the toes to the heel, using the flat of your fist and uncurling your wrist as you move down.

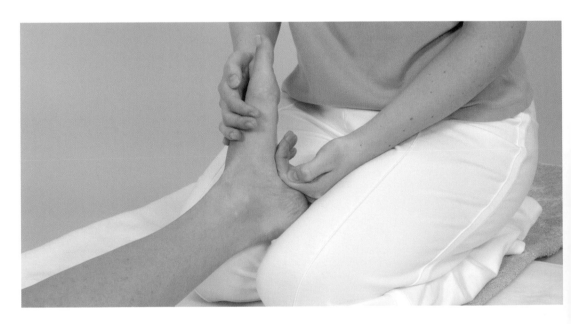

❷ Repeat, covering the full length of the sole of the foot using this fist stroke. Repeat four or five times, applying a little more pressure each time, always working downward.

foot stretch

Work firmly against the resistance of the foot here, taking care not to let your fingers or thumbs slide. Feet are very strong, and you may be surprised at the amount of pressure your partner can withstand.

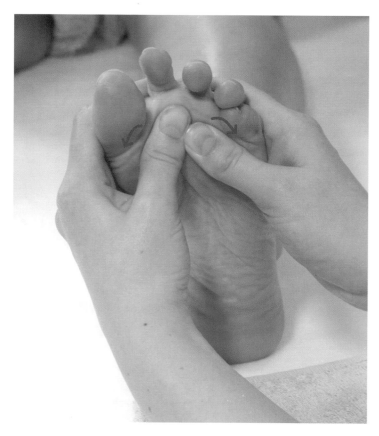

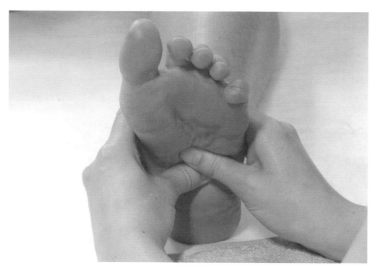

❷ Hold the stretch for 5–8 seconds and release slowly. The beginning and end of the stretch should be performed gradually. Repeat the stretch several times, gradually moving your thumbs down toward the heel.

❶ Place your thumbs one above the other on the arch of the foot. Hold the top of the foot with the fingers of both hands overlapping. Push your thumbs into the sole; at the same time, pull your fingers down, pulling the toes toward the center of the sole to exaggerate the arch of the foot.

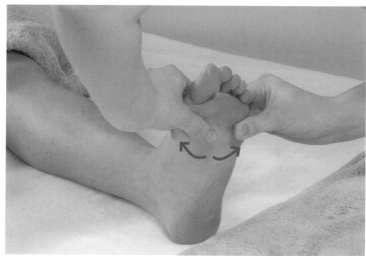

❸ Once you have reached the heel, reverse the action by stretching the foot in the opposite direction. Using your elbows as levers, pull the sides of the foot up and away from the center of the sole, almost as if turning the foot inside out. Repeat slowly several times, back up toward the toes.

toe squeeze

Use this gentle pressure technique to relax tension and improve the range of movement in the toes.

❶ Support the foot with one hand; with the other, squeeze each toe in turn from its base to the tip between your fingers and thumb. Gently pull the toe and release.

❷ Grasp each toe in turn between your fingers and thumb and rotate to increase mobility.

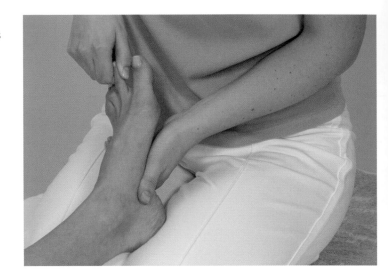

lymph drainage

Being on your feet all day can cause swelling in the feet and ankles because of the accumulation of lymph caused by gravity and poor circulation. This technique helps the drainage of lymph back toward the heart.

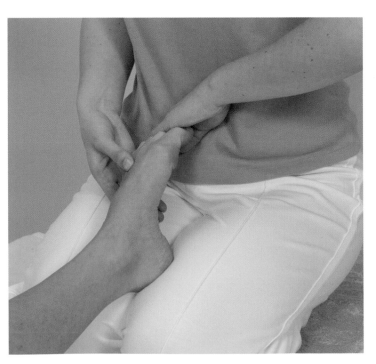

❶ Working on the top of the foot, hold the toes down with one thumb to open up the joints.

❷ Following the gaps between each toe one at a time, trace the spaces between the bones with your other thumb, working up from the toes toward the ankle. Stop when you reach the bridge of the foot. Lift your thumb away from the foot and take it back to its starting position. Repeat the stroke, working along each of the four spaces several times.

other techniques for the feet

- Static pressure on the sole (page 45)
- Rolling pressure on the sole (page 47)
- Friction rub on the sole, top, and sides of the foot (page 56)
- Cross-fiber fanning on the sole (page 52)

effleurage for the spine of the foot

Make these flowing movements firm and confident for maximum relaxation.

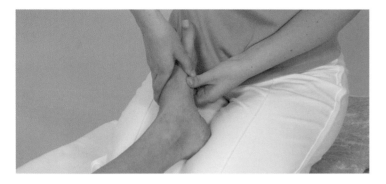

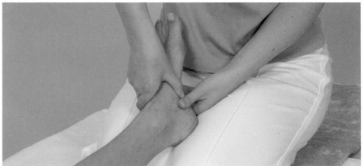

❶ Sandwich the top and sole of the foot between both hands, with your thumbs touching and resting on the outside arch.

❷ Firmly glide both thumbs up the arch toward the ankle, keeping them parallel. Keep the fingers relaxed, trailing beside the thumb in gentle support.

❸ As you approach the ankle, slide the thumbs away from each other, and glide your hands back down toward the toes, ready to repeat the stroke from the beginning.

ankle rub

Finish the massage on this foot by energizing it with a friction rub at the ankle.

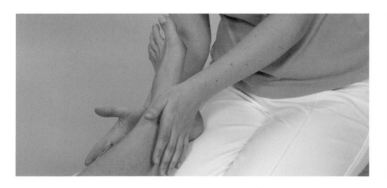

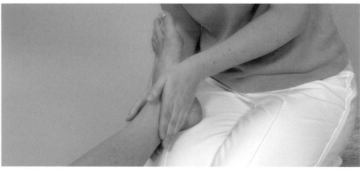

❶ Place the heels of both hands on either side of the foot, just below the ankle.

❷ Rapidly rub the sides of the foot with the heels of your hands alternately, setting up a small but brisk movement. This will have the effect of jostling the foot at the ankle joint.

❸ Repeat all the techniques from page 87 onward on the other foot.

the arms and hands

Not only are the hands and arms often neglected, they are prone to injury at work—from pulled muscles and tennis elbow to the repetitive-strain injuries that come with using the computer. Massage of the arms and hands is important for anyone who use these parts of the body as tools of the trade to ensure that muscular strains are minimized and the likelihood of injury is reduced. Perform all the strokes that follow on one arm and hand, then shift your position to work on the other side.

starting position: Ask your partner to lie on his or her back, and cover well with towels to maintain body temperature. Uncover the arm and shoulder closest to you, and kneel to face your partner. Move the arm away from the rest of the body slightly so you can massage it easily. Apply oil to the whole arm, hand, and around the shoulder. As you work, be careful not to apply pressure over the elbow joint; instead, just glide over the area.

effleurage for the arms

As you soothe the whole region with these calming strokes, keep as much of your hand as possible in contact with your partner's skin.

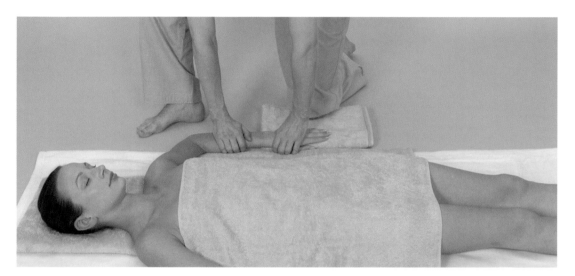

❶ Arrange the arm so that the palm of your partner's hand faces down with the elbow bent and pointing outward so the hand curves in toward the body. Anchor the arm by placing one hand on your partner's hand.

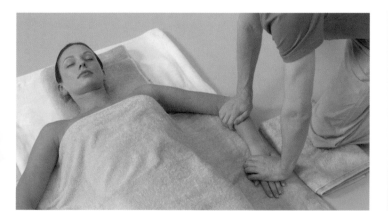

❷ Cup your other hand around the top of the wrist, and slowly stroke it up the length of the arm. Lean in with some body weight and allow your upper body to travel in the direction of the upward stroke. Kneeling on one knee will assist this.

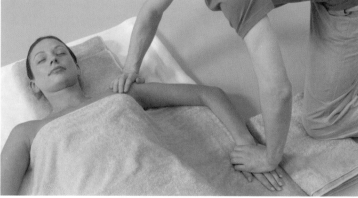

❸ As you reach the shoulder, sweep your hand outward to cover the whole joint, then gently pull your hand back down the outside of the arm, leading with your wrist.

effleurage for the hand

Even with this small action you can use your body movement to help the massage flow. Rocking with the technique makes it hypnotic and relaxing to give.

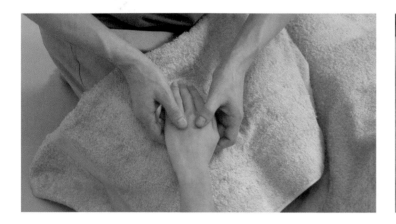 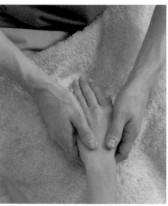 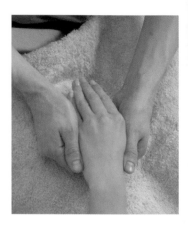

❶ Gently lift your partner's hand off the floor and place it in your lap for support. Sandwich the hand between your hands, with your fingers underneath and thumbs on top.

❷ Using both thumbs simultaneously, slowly stroke up the center of the back of the hand, keeping your thumbs parallel.

❸ Keeping the rhythm and pressure even, as your thumbs reach the wrist joint, sweep them outward around the joint and glide back down the sides of the hand, ready to repeat the movement.

lymph drainage

As the lymphatic system has no pump, massage can assist the flow of lymph toward the lymph ducts, speeding up removal of waste.

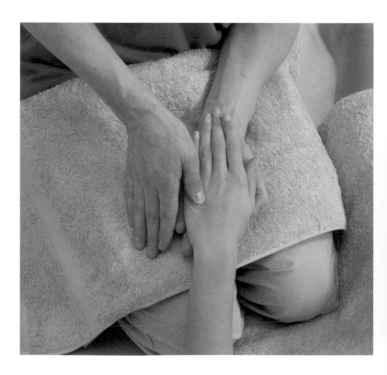

❶ Hold your partner's hand in one of your hands, the back of the hand facing upward.

❷ Using the gaps between each of your partner's fingers as a guide, trace the spaces between the bones with your thumb, stroking up the back of the hand to just below the wrist.

❸ Lift the thumb away from the hand and take it back to the starting position, ready to repeat the stroke. Work along each of the four spaces several times.

circular pressure into the palm

Now rest the back of your partner's hand in yours or place it on your lap.

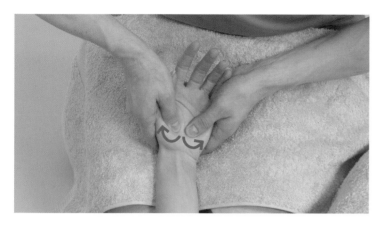 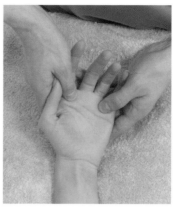 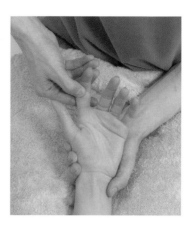

❶ With both thumbs, apply small, deep, circular pressure into the palm of your partner's hand. Concentrate on one spot on the palm, repeating the action several times and rocking into the movement with your body weight.

❷ Apply the technique to a different area of the palm, working in this way until the whole palm has been covered.

❸ Now massage each finger in turn, applying the pressure with one thumb only and working between the joints.

fist stroke

After performing deep, circular pressure work, it feels good to soothe the hand with this repetitive stroke.

❶ Support your partner's hand with one hand, with the fingers pointing toward you. Make a fist with your other hand.

❷ Use your fist to stroke up the length of your partner's palm, from the tips of the fingers to just below the wrist. Lift your hand away and take it back to the starting position, ready to repeat the stroke, keeping your partner's hand supported at all times with your other hand.

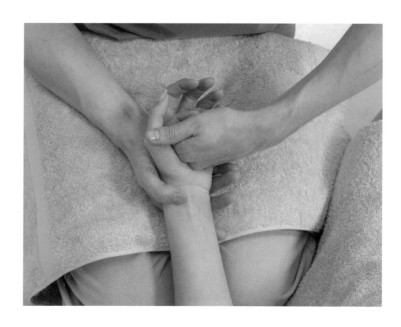

loosening the joints

Move your partner's hand into a relaxed position, supported with the palm facing down.

❶ Take one finger between your thumb and fingers at the point at which it joins the hand. Squeeze and release the sides of the finger several times, working along its length to the tip.

❷ Pause to stroke around the knuckle joints of the fingers with your thumb.

❸ Repeat the squeeze-and-release motion and then the knuckle stroking on each finger in turn.

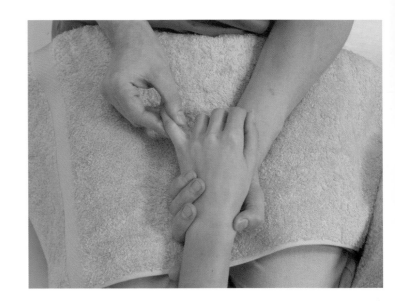

mobilizing the wrists

Keeping your partner's upper arm on the floor, bend the arm at the elbow.

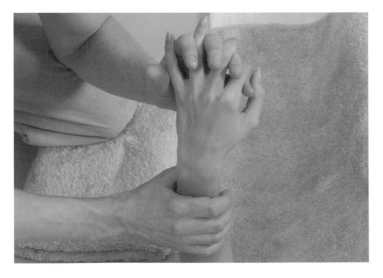

❶ Hold your partner's wrist, and with your other hand, interlock your fingers with your partner's, palm to palm.

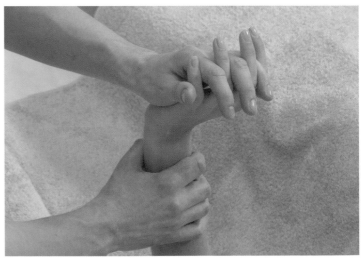

❷ Ensuring your partner's wrist remains still, gently make small circles by rotating your interlocking hands. Work clockwise several times and then repeat, moving counterclockwise.

pulling the fingers

Do not perform this technique if your partner has a tendency toward dislocation of the joints or has arthritis.

Grasp the base of one finger and give it a gentle pull, stretching the finger without causing any pain. Repeat on each finger in turn.

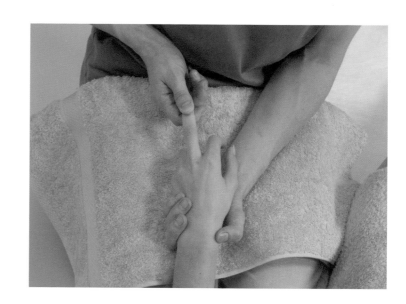

muscle squeeze

Keep your partner's arm in the same position, with your hand still supporting in the same way. Take care to ensure that the wrist and hand are supported at all times during this movement.

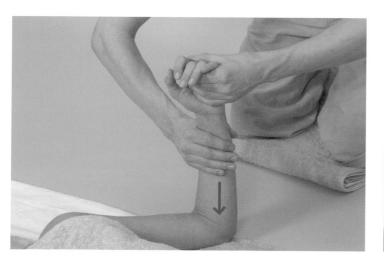

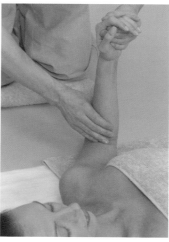

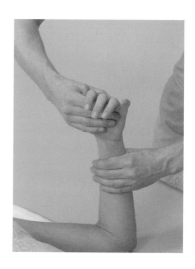

❶ Place the V of your other hand beneath your supporting hand. Use the V to squeeze the muscles down the length of your partner's forearm from wrist to elbow.

❷ When you reach the elbow, glide your fingers back up to the wrist.

❸ Swap hands so the working hand becomes the supporting hand and vice versa. Repeat the muscle-squeeze action on the other side of your partner's arm. Work once again from wrist to elbow.

transverse pressure

As you work on this technique, you may notice a slight uncurling of the fingers as you approach the elbow; this is a reflex action and is quite normal.

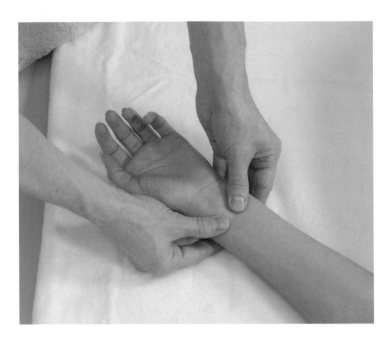

❶ Replace the arm gently on the floor. Place both your thumbs, tip to tip, immediately above your partner's wrist. Rest your fingers lightly on the back of his or her arm.

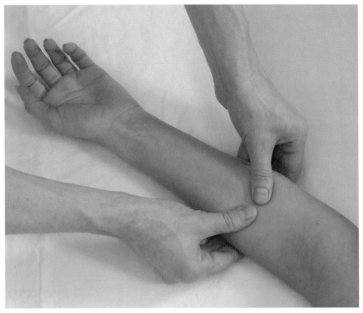

❷ Glide your thumbs together down the middle of the forearm, maintaining an even and constant pressure as you move toward the elbow. Release the pressure as you approach the elbow joint.

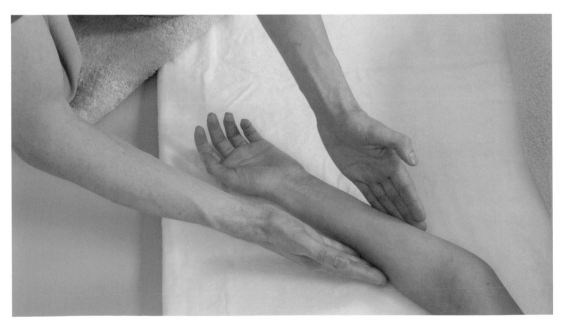

❸ With fingers and thumbs together, glide your hand back up the sides of the arm. Use your body weight to apply pressure on the downward stroke, and lift it away on the upward stroke.

fist stroking

Never apply pressure over the elbow area with this stroke; simply glide over the joint. Your nonworking hand should support your partner's wrist at all times.

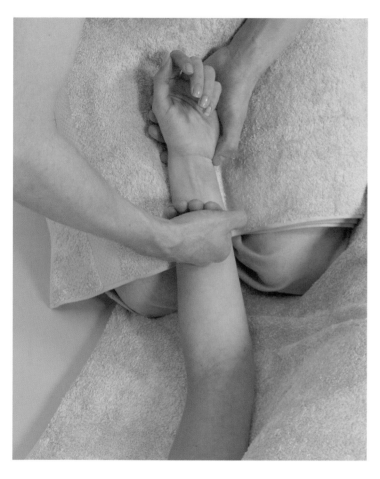

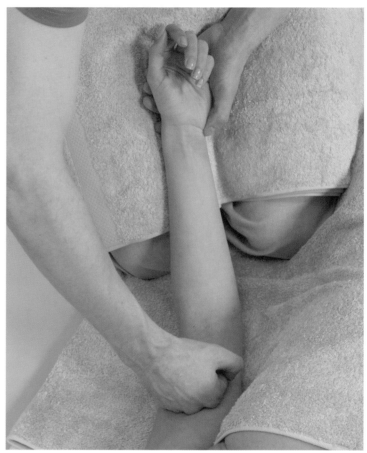

❶ Place your partner's arm in your lap, palm turned upward. Gently hold his or her wrist with one hand, keeping a slight bend in the elbow. Make a fist with your other hand and place the flat of the fist just above the wrist joint.

❷ Let the fist travel from wrist to elbow, applying steady and firm pressure. Release the pressure just before you reach the elbow joint.

❸ Glide your fist lightly over the elbow joint and reintroduce pressure into the stroke along the length of the upper arm, moving toward the shoulder. Lift your fist away as you approach the shoulder joint. Return your fist to the starting position, just above the wrist joint, ready to begin again.

arm stretch

Urge your partner to let go of control in this series of passive stretches, allowing you to make all the movements.

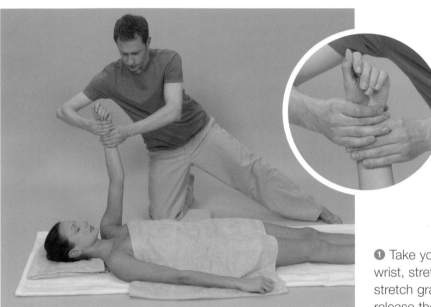

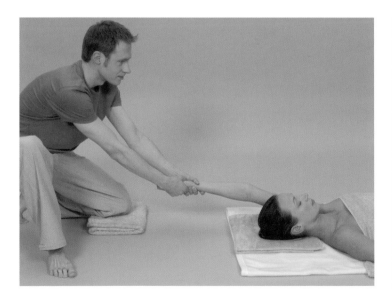

1 Take your partner's nearest arm, and supporting it at the wrist, stretch it gently up toward the ceiling. Move into the stretch gradually and hold it for 8–10 seconds. Slowly release the stretch.

2 Still supporting the arm, take it back behind your partner's head. Stretch the limb as before, then slowly release.

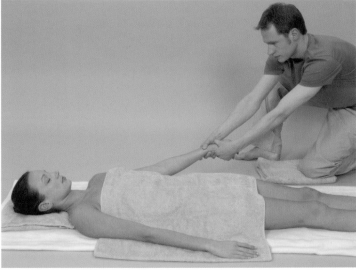

3 Complete the series of stretches by taking the supported arm back to your partner's side and slowly stretching the limb toward the toes.

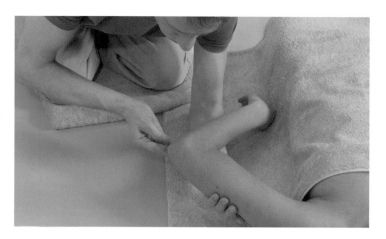

elbow stroking

The skin around the elbow joint tends to be dry, and massaging oil into the area helps combat any roughness.

Raise your partner's arm to allow the elbow to point outward. Circle around the elbow with your fingertips, using firm contact to prevent ticklishness.

muscle rolling

Now replace your partner's arm on the floor, palm facing downward and arm slightly bent at the elbow.

❶ Create a triangle with the thumbs and index fingers of both hands and place this on your partner's biceps at the front of the upper arm.

❷ Grasp the biceps between your fingers and thumbs, and roll the muscle with your thumbs toward your fingers, keeping the fingers still. Repeat the movement several times.

❸ Repeat the rolling action over the entire muscle area of the upper arm, including on the triceps at the back of the arm.

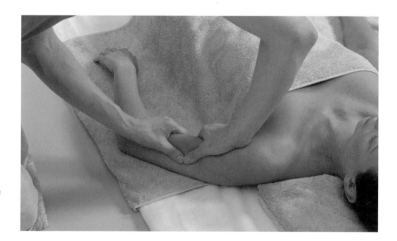

finishing touches

Complete the massage with a soothing effleurage before turning your attention to the other arm.

❶ Follow the soothing effleurage routine again from page 95.

❷ Move to the other side of the body to repeat the massage from page 95 onward on the other arm and hand.

other techniques for the arms and hands

- Rolling pressure on any tight muscles (page 47)
- Combing all over (page 49)
- Raking all over (page 49)
- Raindrops all over (page 51)
- Cross-fiber fanning on the biceps and triceps (page 52)
- Circling all over (page 53)
- Feathering down the length of the arm (page 56)

the abdomen

There are huge benefits to receiving an abdomen massage: it can help balance the digestive system, calming an overactive digestion and stimulating a sluggish one. Many people hold tension in the abdomen, particularly women in search of that elusive flat tummy. Stress seems to target the abdomen, aggravating disorders such as irritable bowel syndrome, constipation, and indigestion. Massage can help alleviate the symptoms. Some people may be a little reluctant to have an abdomen massage, but, once experienced, they often become lifelong fans.

CAUTION: Massage the abdomen in a clockwise direction (the direction of digestion) and work with care, as many organs underlie the abdominal muscles.

starting position: Ask your partner to lie on his or her back, then cover with towels to retain warmth. Use two separate towels to enable you to keep the upper and lower body warm, and uncover your partner's abdomen only.

starting the massage
To introduce yourself and the massage to your partner, make sure you let him or her know when you are about to begin.

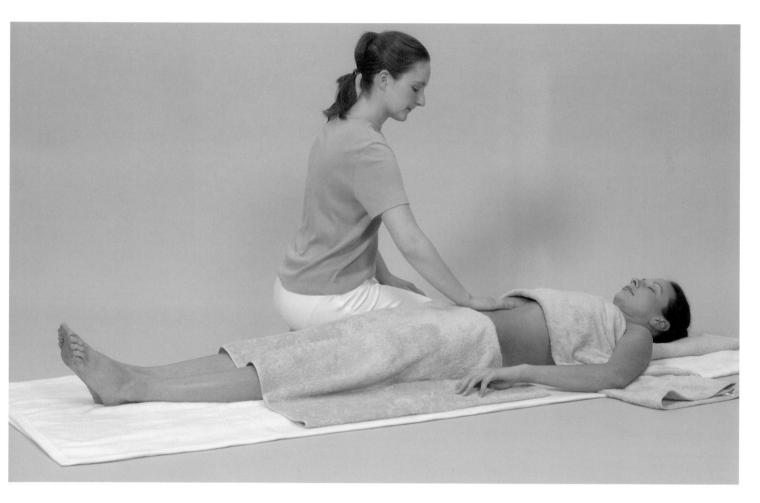

❶ Position yourself at your partner's side, facing the head. Place one hand slowly over the navel and rest it there for a while to reduce sensitivity.

❷ Keeping one hand in contact with the skin, apply oil to the whole abdomen, making the strokes firm and even to prevent ticklishness.

effleurage for the abdomen

Make your strokes confident, building up a smooth rhythm to reassure your partner.

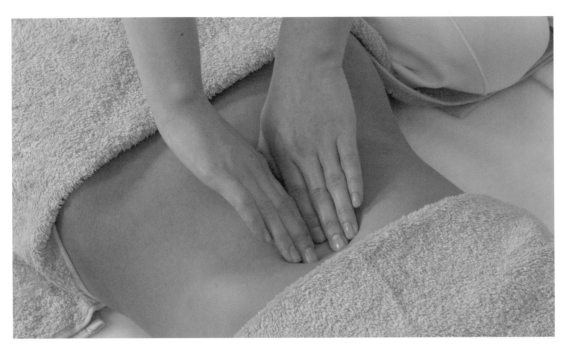

❶ Position your hands so your fingers point toward your partner's head. Glide both hands simultaneously up the center of the abdomen, as far as the third or fourth rib. To make your position more comfortable, lift your outer fingers and tilt your hands inward as you reach the rib cage so that your thumbs and index and middle fingers can sweep up the center of the hollow.

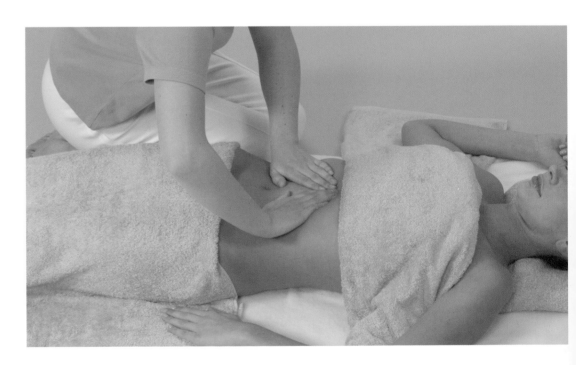

❷ Glide back down the abdomen, allowing your hands to turn out and away from each other to stroke beneath the ribs on either side of the abdomen. Be careful with the amount of pressure you use, especially if your partner has recently eaten.

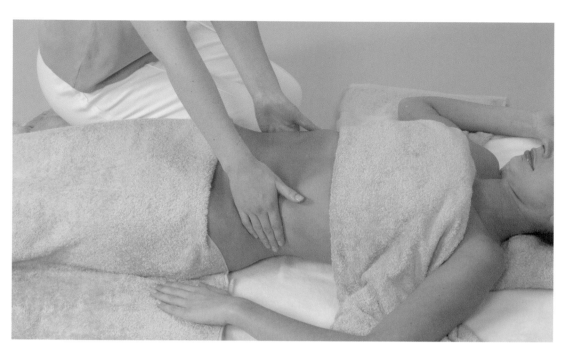

3 Turn your hands 180 degrees so that, once again, your fingers point outward, and take your hands behind your partner's back, bringing the fingertips of both hands to touch.

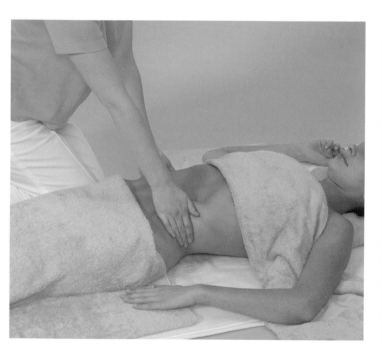

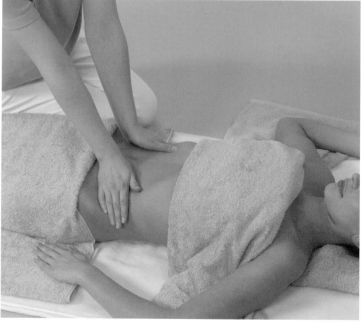

4 Leading with the wrists, start to bring your hands back toward the front of the body, pulling your hands back toward each other firmly as if trying to reduce your partner's waistline. To assist, use your own body weight to increase the pull.

5 Allow the abdominal muscles to release gradually from your hands and relax your own body. To complete the effleurage, sweep your hands in to just below the navel, ready to repeat the whole movement several times.

thumb tracing

Allow the thumbs to lead this light movement.

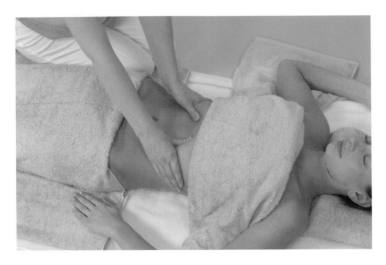

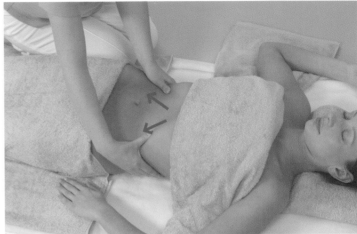

❶ Place your thumbs next to each other just beneath the rib cage at the bottom of your partner's breastbone. Stretch your fingers away from your thumbs slightly and rest them lightly on your partner's sides.

❷ Trace your thumbs out beneath the ribs toward your partner's sides. Let your fingers glide lightly as your thumbs lead outward. With fingers and thumbs together, sweep your hands back in toward the center, ready to repeat the stroke.

solar plexus stroke

This is a light (but not ticklish) movement. The solar plexus is a dense cluster of nerve cells that control vital functions such as the secretion of adrenaline.

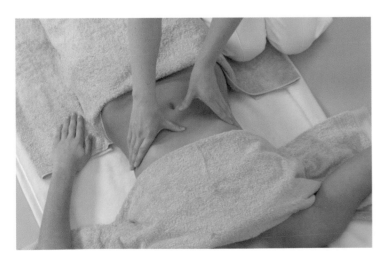

❶ Position one thumb just below the breastbone where the lower ribs join it, and gently stroke upward into the hollow, lifting the thumb as you pass over the bone.

❷ Repeat the stroke with the other thumb as the first thumb lifts off, completing about six or eight strokes in total.

circular pressure

Shift your position slightly so that you face your partner's abdomen. As you massage, make sure that the end of one circular movement links to the beginning of the next.

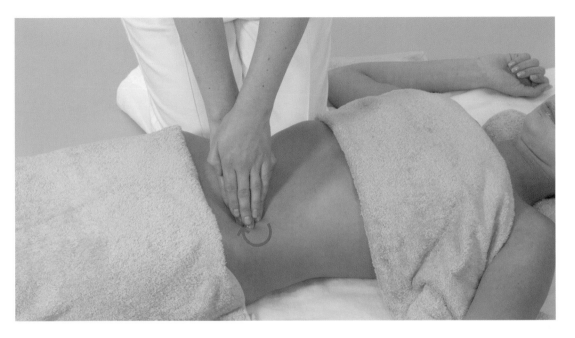

❶ Place the fingertips of one hand on top of the other at the bottom of the descending colon. Beginning a few finger-widths away from the navel, apply small, deep, circular pressures, working over one spot several times.

❷ Remaining in contact with your partner's skin, glide your fingers 1–2 inches or so and repeat the stroke, gradually progressing around the whole abdominal area in a clockwise direction.

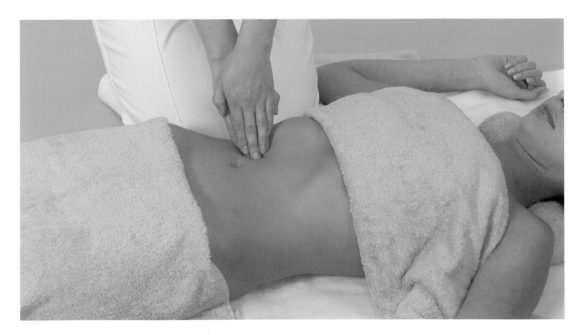

alternate circling

Ensure that the lifting off and putting on of your second hand is a gentle, not sudden, movement here, continuing the flow as you repeat the technique over and over again.

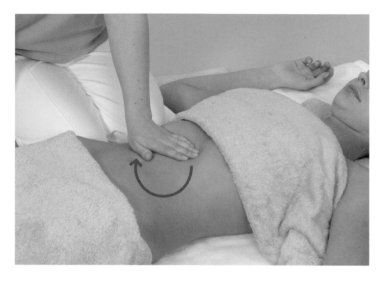

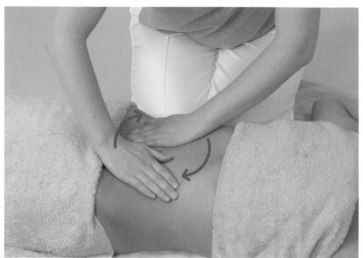

❶ Stroke the whole abdominal area in one big clockwise circle with the palm of your left hand. This hand circles continuously, slowly, and steadily throughout the movement.

❷ Let your right hand also make large stroking circles on the abdomen in a clockwise direction at the same speed and following the left hand so that the movements flow together.

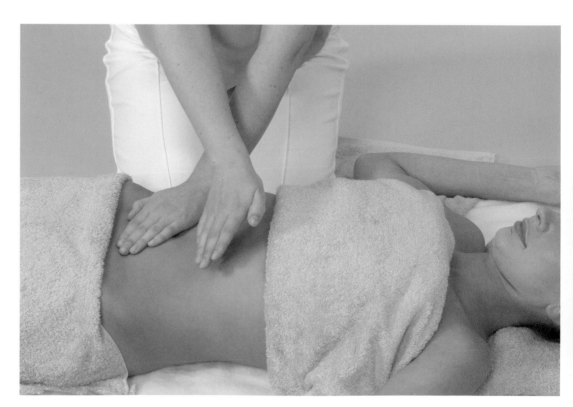

❸ Just before the hands cross, lift your right hand over your left hand, returning it to the abdomen to complete its circle. Repeat over and over, keeping the lifting away and replacing of the right hand gentle and steady so as not to interrupt the flow of the movement.

alternate kneading

Once you become confident with this technique, you will develop a natural rhythm that allows your own body weight and movement to make the action more effective.

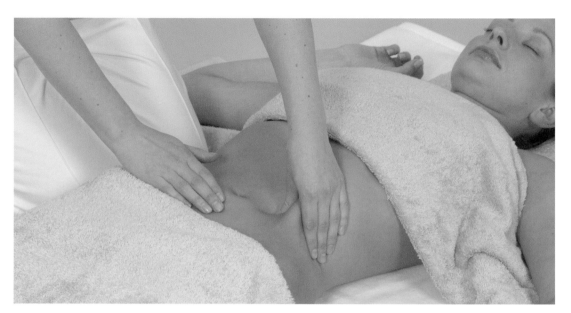

❶ Place one hand on your partner's side (the side furthest away from you), thumb on the abdomen and fingers stretched away from you. Using the V of this hand, grasp the muscle between your fingers and thumb. Use the fingers to pull the muscle back toward the thumb.

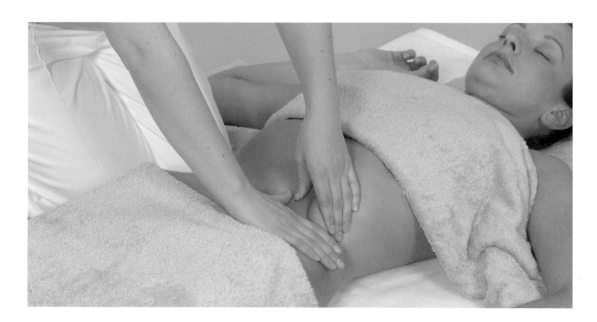

❷ Just before this first hand finishes the kneading movement, repeat the manipulation of the muscles on the same side of the abdomen using your other hand.

❸ Repeat this alternate-hands action several times, then move around to your partner's other side and repeat the whole technique.

push and pull

This technique feels like the ebb and flow of waves on a beach and is very satisfying to both give and receive. Rock your body to assist the push-and-pull motion.

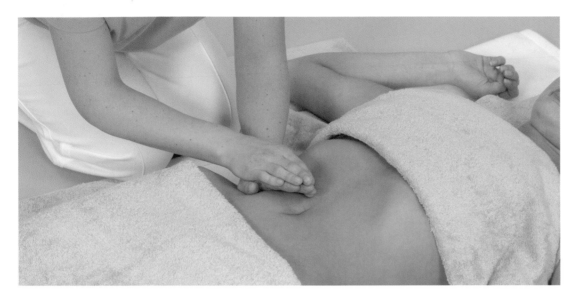

❶ Kneel facing your partner's abdomen. Place both hands on the near side of the waist, with your fingers pointing away from you.

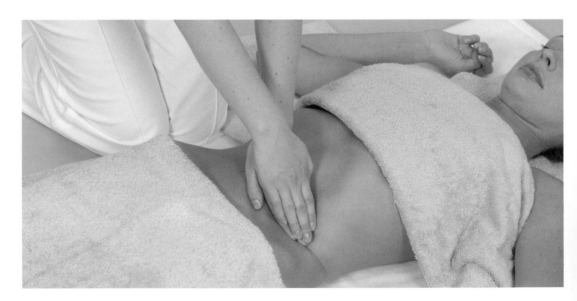

❷ Using the heel of your hands as much as possible, lift the tissue on the side of the waist and hip and push it over to the center of the abdomen, gliding your hands in that direction.

❸ Release the pushing motion, allowing the emphasis of the movement to pass to your fingertips, which grasp the tissue on the other side of the waist and other hip. Pull the tissue here toward you, then release, ready to repeat the pushing movement again.

one thousand hands

This effleurage movement should be performed very slowly as a conclusion to an abdomen massage sequence.

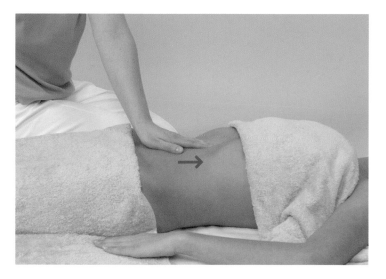

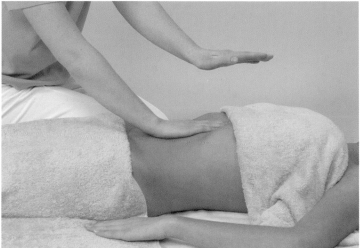

❶ Position yourself at your partner's side, level with the hips, facing up the body. Gently place the flat of one hand, fingers and thumbs parallel and touching, onto the center of the lower abdomen.

❸ As the first hand lifts away, glide your other hand up the center of your partner's abdomen to repeat the stroke. Keep one hand moving upward on your partner's abdomen at all times, so that it feels like one continuous movement. To help your posture and the pressure of the stroke, rock forward with each upward stroke.

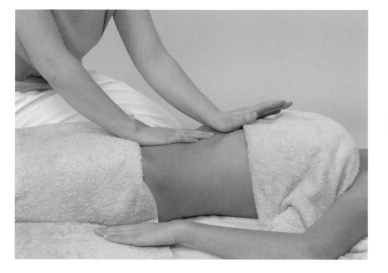

❷ Glide your hand slowly up the center of the abdomen as far as the base of the ribs. As this first hand nears the base of the ribs, begin to lift the fingers up, keeping the heel of the hand in contact with the skin as you place your other hand on the center of the lower abdomen.

other techniques for the abdomen

- Static pressure in a clockwise circle around the intestines (page 45)
- Wringing across the width of the abdomen (page 48)
- Combing across the width of the abdomen (page 49)
- Circling in a clockwise direction with one hand (page 53)
- Friction rub just below the navel (page 56)

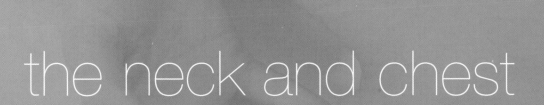

> Develop contact between yourself and your body—that temple in which you live.
>
> **Virginia Satir**

the neck and chest

The neck is an area of the body particularly prone to holding tension. This is not always caused by stress; neck muscles have to work hard to keep the head upright throughout our waking hours. A neck massage, therefore, can be absolute heaven. Although you will find some massage techniques for the neck incorporated into the back sequence (from page 61 onward), it is wonderful to dedicate a whole massage to the neck and chest.

starting position: Ask your partner to lie on his or her back, then cover with towels to maintain warmth. Position yourself behind your partner's head, and uncover the shoulders and top of the chest, respecting modesty for a woman.

nudging

Many of us definitely have room for improvement when it comes to posture, and it is common to have an inclination toward being round-shouldered and to have the shoulders lifted. Work on the chest to release tension in the pectoral muscles can go some way to rectifying this.

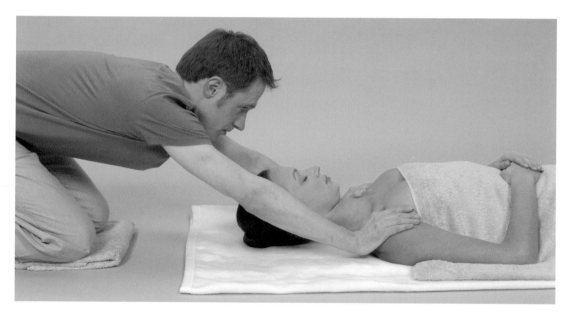

❶ Place one hand on each of your partner's shoulders, fingers pointing outward.

❷ Lean over the body and gradually increase the amount of body weight you apply to one shoulder to encourage it to relax toward the feet. Hold for 10–20 seconds before slowly releasing and repeating on the other side.

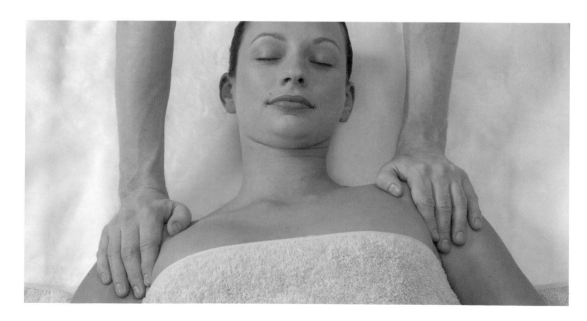

effleurage for the chest, neck, and shoulders

Because the neck muscles are so strong, they can usually withstand substantial pressure—but do ask your partner for feedback. Keep checking that your thumbs are away from the throat as you massage.

❶ Apply oil to the chest, neck, and shoulder area with broad, sweeping strokes. With fingers and thumbs together and pointing inward, place your hands, palms down, on the center of your partner's chest, just below the collarbone.

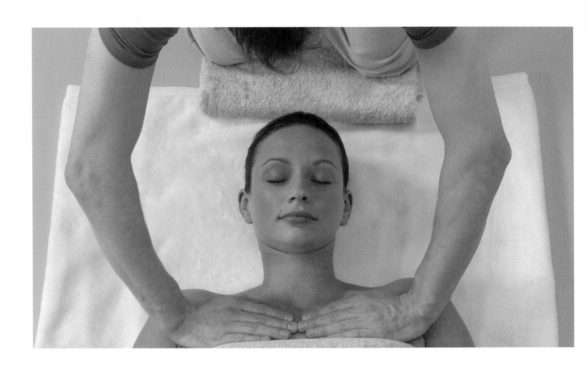

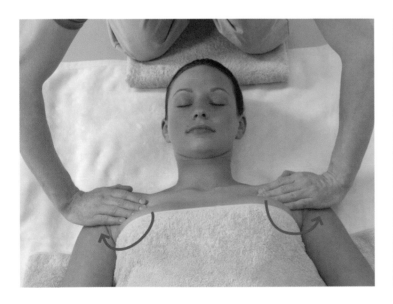

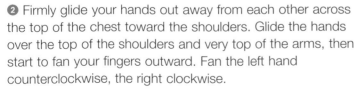

❷ Firmly glide your hands out away from each other across the top of the chest toward the shoulders. Glide the hands over the top of the shoulders and very top of the arms, then start to fan your fingers outward. Fan the left hand counterclockwise, the right clockwise.

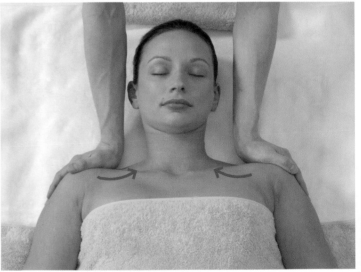

❸ With fingers now pointing outward, cup your hands around the contours of your partner's shoulders. Using pressure mainly from your fingertips on the underneath of the shoulders, pull along the shoulder muscle with strong, rigid fingers, moving in toward the neck.

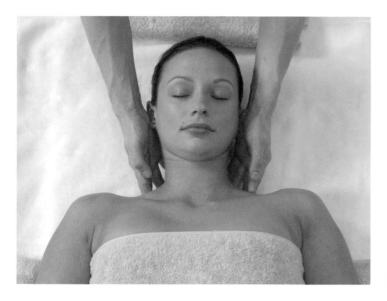

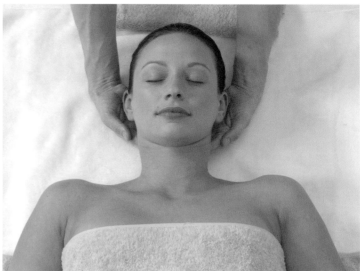

❹ Still applying most pressure with the fingers, draw your hands up the back of the neck, pulling the muscles with you. Use your body weight to assist this part of the massage.

❺ As you reach the nape of the neck, draw your fingertips up to the base of the skull, leaning back to add a little stretch as the fingers pull on the back of the skull.

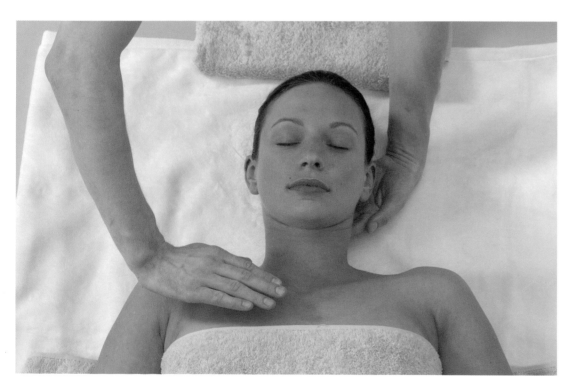

❻ Lift one hand off the back of the neck and place it in its original position on the top of the chest, followed by the other hand, ready to repeat the stroke. This ensures that you maintain contact with your partner while avoiding the throat.

alternating effleurage

This movement is similar to the last stroke, the variation being that one hand performs the technique, followed by the other. This establishes a gentle swaying motion for your partner to relax into.

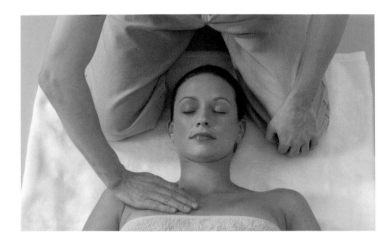

❶ Place one palm horizontally across the top of your partner's chest, just below the collarbone. Glide your hand away from the breastbone, wrist leading, across the top of the chest and around the shoulder.

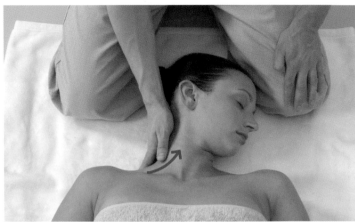

❸ As your hand moves up the neck, encourage the head to roll to the side with a gentle nudge of the forearm.

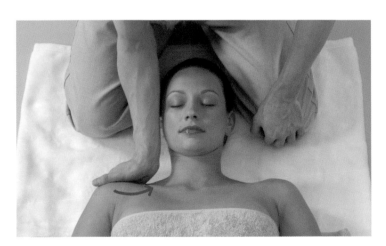

❷ With the wrist still leading, firmly glide your hand over the trapezius muscle at the back of the shoulder and bring it up the side of the neck.

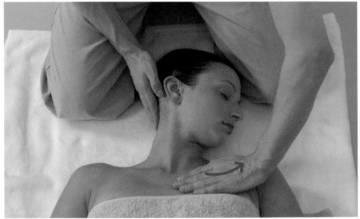

❹ Applying firm finger pressure, draw your fingers up the side of the neck, pulling into the muscles. Pull all the way into the base of the skull by the hairline. As this first hand completes the movement, place your other hand on the top of the chest, ready to repeat the stroke on the other side.

❺ Repeat, alternating hands with each stroke and swaying with the technique to set up a gentle rhythm.

deep stroking

Ensure you finish the previous movement with your partner's head turned to the left, then move straight on to this technique. As one hand is in contact with your partner's head at all times, it is acceptable to lose contact with your working hand.

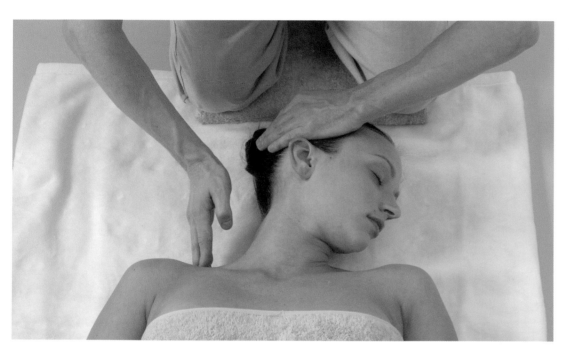

❶ Keep the head steady with your left hand to prevent it from rolling. Place your right hand, palm upward, beneath your partner's right shoulder, with the head turned away.

❷ Stroke firmly with your fingertips up the back of the shoulder. Apply a great deal of pressure on this upward stroke, using your body weight to help you pull up.

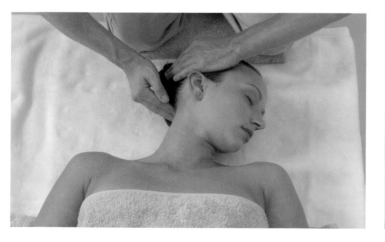

❸ Continue the stroke up the side of the neck, increasing the pressure until you reach the hairline. Rhythmically release your contact, taking your hand back to the starting position to repeat the stroke. After repeating several times, begin to lighten the touch.

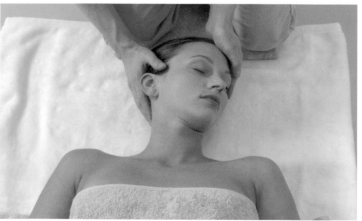

❹ Carefully and slowly roll the head to the other side, using both hands to guide its weight. Then perform the technique on the other side of the neck using your other hand.

double-handed pull-up

This technique is made effective by the counterweight of your partner's body against your pressure.

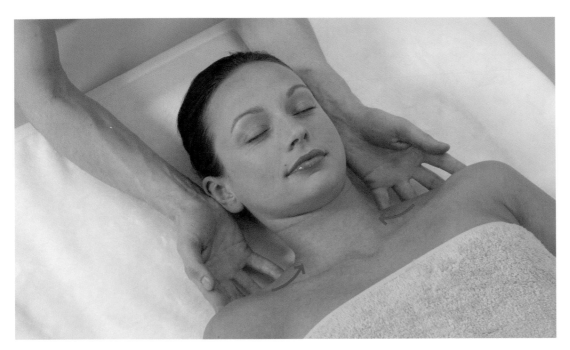

❶ Slowly roll your partner's head back into a central position. Crouching down low, rest your forearms on the floor, palms facing upward and fingertips in contact with the underside and outer edge of each shoulder.

❷ Splay your fingers so that they point upward, and press into the shoulders. Pull strongly into the back of the shoulders toward the center of the body.

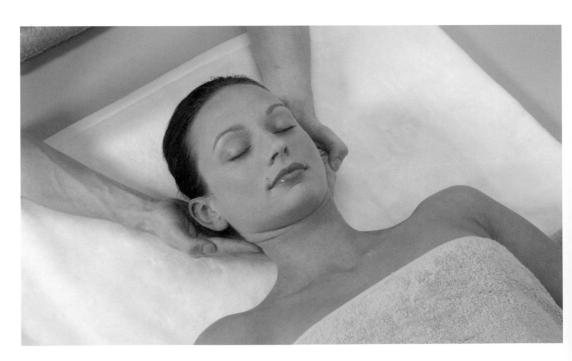

❸ Continue pulling up the back of the neck, fingers on either side of the cervical spine in the neck. Lean back as your fingers pull, lifting your partner's head slightly away from the floor to stretch the neck gently.

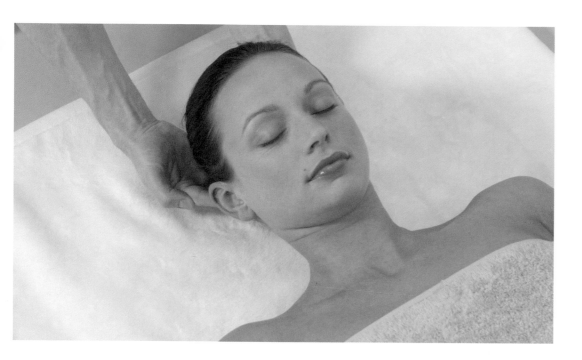

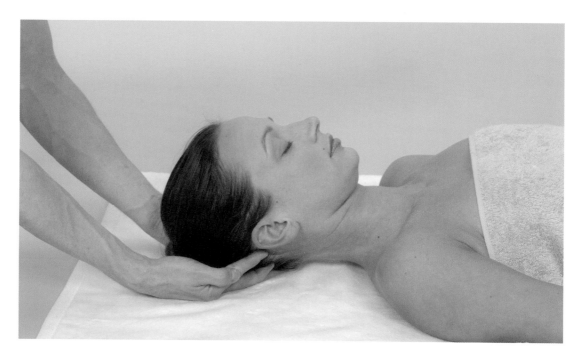

❹ When you reach the base of the skull, delicately pull through the hair, release the head gently, and repeat the whole movement in a rhythmical fashion.

neck stretch

Mobility in the neck is vital for quality of life—have you ever tried to reverse a car with a stiff neck? To boost mobility, it's useful to incorporate a stretch into a neck-massage sequence.

❶ Keeping the head rolled to one side, shift position to sit by the side of your partner's neck.

❷ With one hand on the shoulder and one on the head, slowly and carefully pull your hands apart to elongate the neck. Move slowly and ask for feedback to ensure that the stretch remains comfortable. Your partner should feel a pull, but no pain.

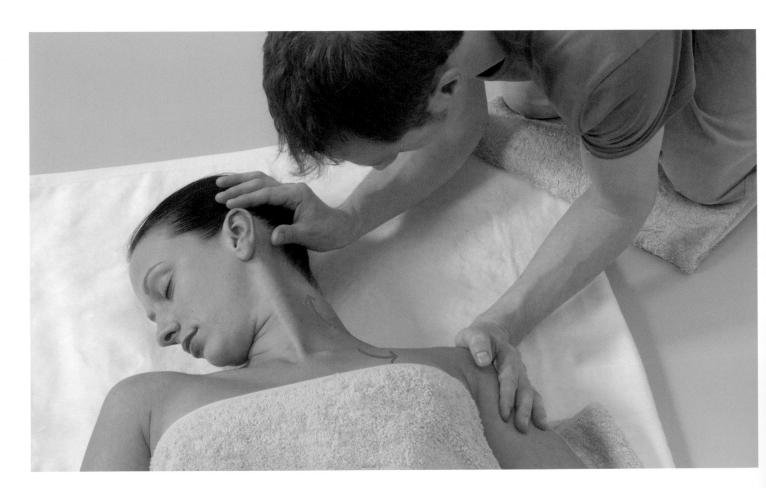

❸ Move around your partner's body to repeat the stretch on the other side of the neck.

head rolls

Kneel behind your partner's head. The slowness of this movement is what makes it relaxing. Keep the hand supporting the head in contact with the floor throughout the move.

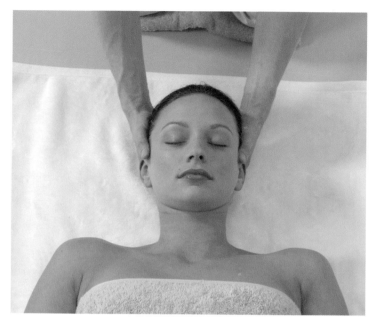

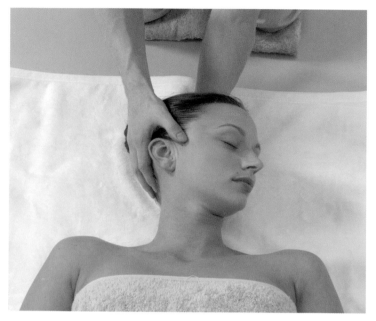

❶ With fingers and thumbs together, slide your hands beneath each side of your partner's head, fingers pointing down toward the back. Be careful not to pull the hair.

❷ With one hand, slowly roll the head to one side, using your other hand as a pivot to assist the turn. Ensure the action is slow and smooth and stays within your partner's normal range of movement.

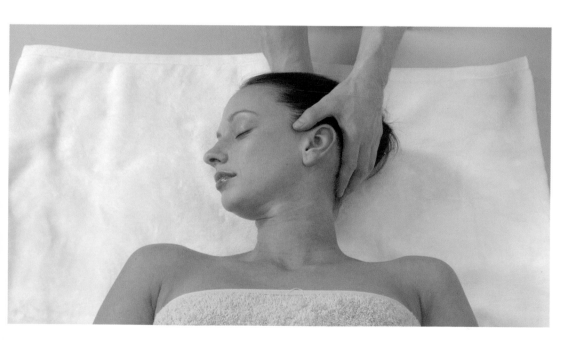

❸ Once the head has gone as far as it can, reverse the action with your other hand to roll the head to the other side; again, ensure that the head is supported at all times. Repeat several times, allowing your body to sway to assist the rolling motion.

fist pressure

Provided you avoid the breasts, you can perform this technique as firmly on women as on men.

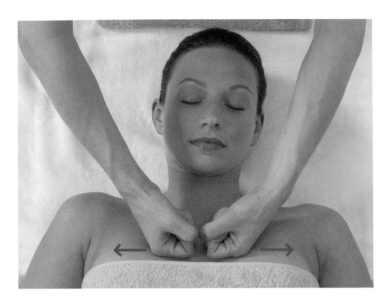

❶ Ensure your partner's head is positioned centrally. Create loose fists with your hands and place the back of the hands horizontally at the top of your partner's chest, knuckles in contact with the pectoral muscles below the collarbone on either side of the breastbone.

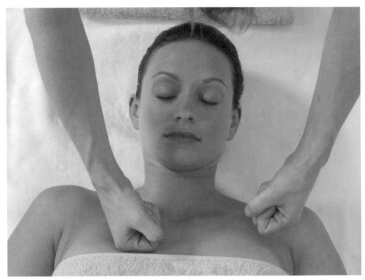

❸ As your fists approach the shoulders, turn them away from you toward each armpit to assist lymphatic drainage. When you reach the armpits, lift one fist, then the other, back to the starting position, ready to repeat the movement.

❹ On men, continue to work down the chest and torso as far as the bottom of the rib cage. Take care when working over the ribs by loosening your hand and combing between the ribs (page 49). Lift each hand in turn away and back to the starting position at the top of the chest to repeat.

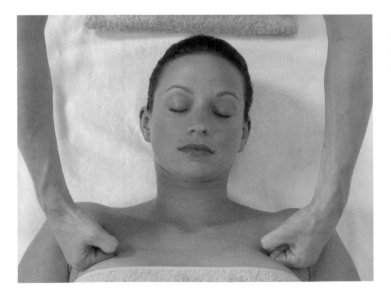

❷ Working outward, firmly glide your fists over the top of the chest toward the shoulders.

tracing the collarbone

Here, the fingers and thumb of each hand squeeze on either side of the collarbone, starting close to the breastbone.

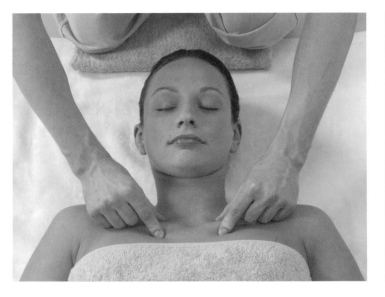

❶ Using both hands, place the thumbs above the collarbone and the fingers below the collarbone at the center of the chest.

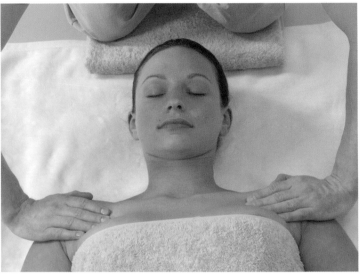

❸ As your hands approach the shoulders, flatten the hands out to glide around the top of the arms and beneath the shoulders.

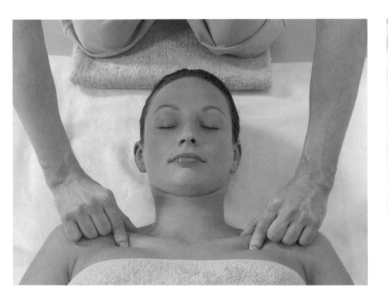

❷ Maintaining pressure, firmly trace the length of each collarbone between your fingers and thumbs by moving your hands outward.

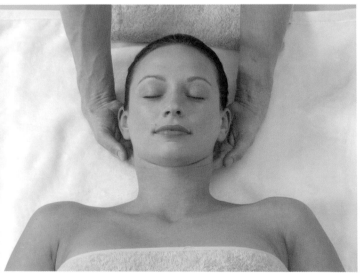

❹ Glide up the neck, then gently lift one hand, and then the other, back to the starting position (always keep one hand in contact with the body), replacing your fingers and thumbs on the collarbone, ready to repeat the movement.

alternate kneading on the pectorals

Build up a smooth rhythm, the movement of one hand imperceptibly flowing into that of the next. Don't rush the movement, as this will reduce the effectiveness of the manipulation.

❶ Taking care to avoid the breasts, place one hand on the pectoral muscles, close to the armpit. Grasp a small amount of muscle between fingers and thumb.

❷ Pull the muscle with your fingers back toward the thumb, allowing it to slip out of your grasp gradually.

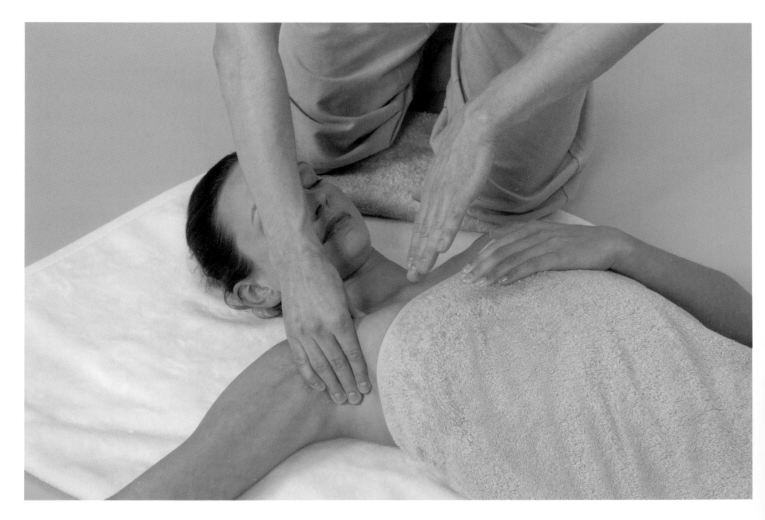

❸ As this first hand completes the movement, let the other hand start the movement over the same muscle. Keep the rhythm smooth, one hand following the other. Repeat on the other side.

❹ Finish by repeating the effleurage strokes on page 116.

scalp massage

To complete the chest and neck sequence, it is pleasant to pay some attention to the head. Most of us unknowingly hold tension in the scalp; this technique really helps release it.

❶ With hands cupped as if holding a ball and fingers strong, make contact with the head using both hands. Form a strong contact between the tips of the fingers and the skin of the scalp.

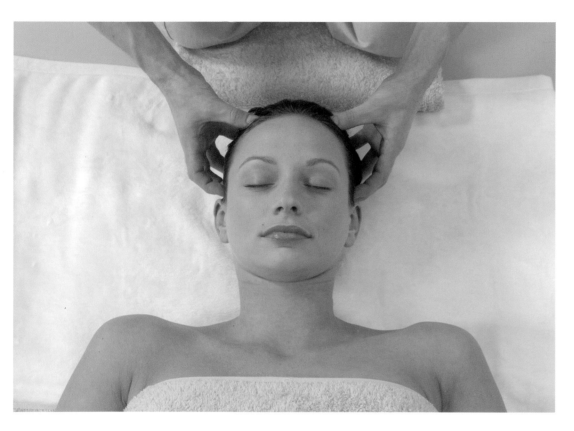

❷ Using your own body weight and movement, rock your body as you circle your hands to manipulate the skin of the scalp. The hair should not move or rustle; this is a strong movement of the scalp to ease tightness and tension.

other techniques for the chest, neck, and shoulders

- Static pressure on the sides of the neck and just below the collarbone (page 45)
- Traveling pressure on the sides of the neck (page 46)
- Rolling pressure on the sides of the neck (page 47)
- Combing on the sides of the neck and across the chest (page 49)
- Cross-fiber fanning on the sides of the neck (page 52)
- Feathering (page 56)

the face

The face can hold as much tension as any other part of the body and deserves some pampering care and attention to ease frown lines, relax tired eyes, and release a tight jaw. The stimulation massage helps circulation, helps the complexion glow, and the nutrients in the oil applied to help your fingertips glide over the face are particularly beneficial for the skin. Try apricot kernel for sensitive or mature skin, evening primrose for dry skin, and jojoba for oily skin, adding wheat-germ oil to create an especially nurturing skin-care blend.

starting position: Ask your partner to lie on his or her back, covered with towels to keep warm. Position yourself behind your partner's head or with his or her head in your lap. With gentle, even strokes, apply a very small amount of oil to the face and neck.

facial relaxation

This simple exercise can ease the frown lines caused by stress even before you start to stroke the face.

❶ Ask your partner to close his or her eyes and breathe slowly and deeply to invoke a state of relaxation.

❷ Cup your hands, fingers, and thumbs together, and gently place them over your partner's face, on either side of the nose. Hold the position for 20–30 seconds while taking slow, deep breaths and using the time to connect with your partner.

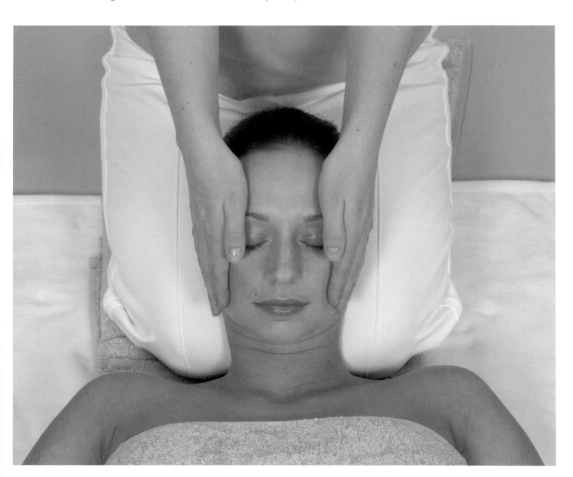

effleurage for the face

Keep this movement gentle and flowing.

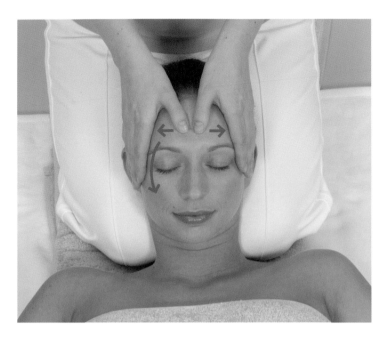

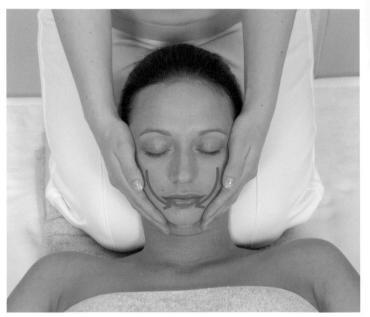

❶ Place both thumbs, gently touching, on your partner's forehead. Allow your fingers to cup around the outside of your partner's temples.

❷ Using your thumbs, firmly stroke outward across the forehead toward the temples. Allow your fingers to glide rhythmically down the outside of the face to the chin.

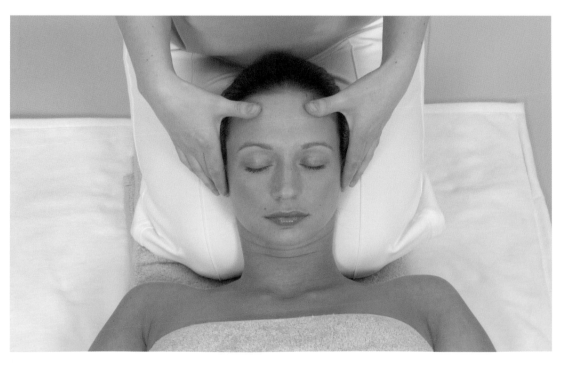

❸ Glide your hands back up the sides of the face to meet, thumbs together, at the center of the forehead. You are now back at the starting position, ready to repeat. Continue several times, building up a smooth, flowing motion. Finish with your hands on the forehead.

effleurage for the forehead

In this stroke you work with alternate hands.

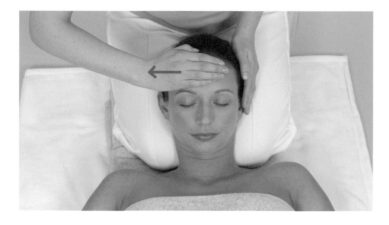

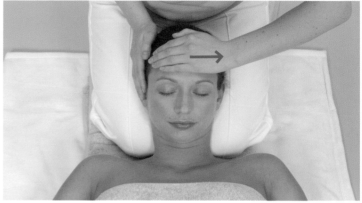

❶ Place the heel of one hand on one side of your partner's forehead, fingers pointing away from the head. Keeping the fingers and thumb together, gently stroke, with the wrist leading, across the width of the forehead to the opposite side.

❷ As you are about to lift away this first hand from the forehead, repeat the stroke in the opposite direction with your other hand. Build up a repetitive flow of alternating hands, allowing your body to flow with the rhythm of the movement.

waterwheel effleurage

This technique is named after the ever-flowing movement of the paddles of a waterwheel. Continue to work in the same rhythmic way as before.

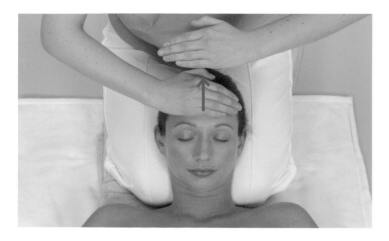

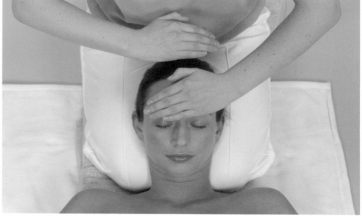

❶ With fingers and thumb together, place one hand lightly across your partner's forehead. Stroke the entire hand from the forehead back toward the hairline.

❷ As you are about to lift away the first hand, repeat the action with the other hand, creating an alternating circle of hands above your partner's head.

stroking around the eyes

Make sure not to drag the delicate skin in this area and to use a very light pressure.

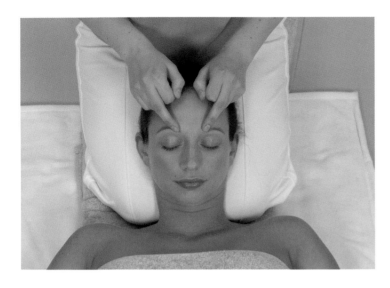

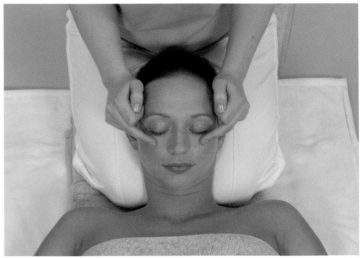

❶ Following the direction of eyebrow growth, start to circle around the eye area with one or two fingers, keeping your touch very light.

❷ Use the bone around the eye socket and the bridge of the nose as your guide.

pressure points on the brow bone

Working on the pressure point at the outer corner of the eye can be of benefit for someone suffering from a headache. Take care to stay clear of the eyes as you work.

❶ Using your index fingers, gently and carefully press just beneath the brow bone of each eye, starting beside the nose. Hold the pressure for a few seconds.

❷ Gently lift the fingers off, move them a little further away from the nose, and repeat the pressure. Continue in five or six places as you gradually move outward across each brow bone, finishing at the outer corner of each eye.

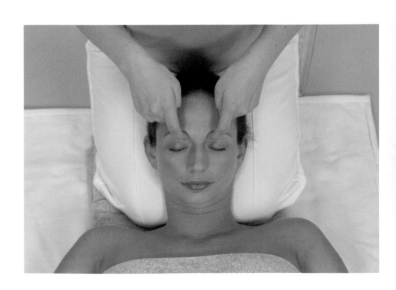

pressure points on the cheekbone

This technique can be beneficial for people with blocked sinuses.

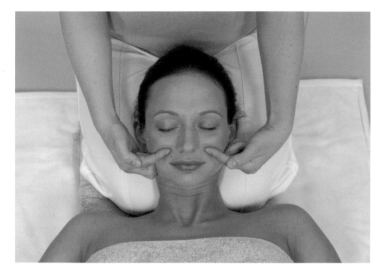

❶ Place the fingertips of each hand beneath the cheekbones, starting beside the nose. Carefully and gently apply pressure upward into the bone. Hold the pressure for a few seconds.

❷ Gently lift the fingers off, move them a little way along the cheekbone away from the nose, and repeat the pressure. Continue applying pressure, working along the cheekbone from the nose to the outside of the face.

eyebrow pinch

This squeeze and release technique feels really invigorating.

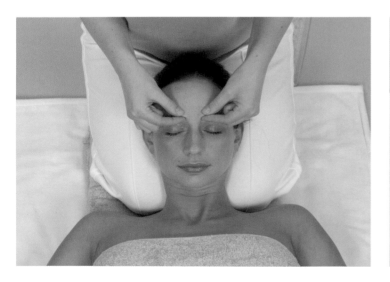

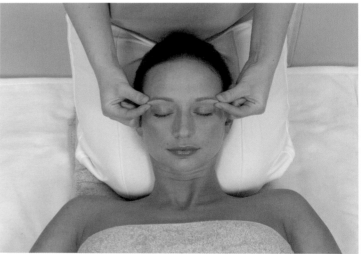

❶ Starting on either side of the bridge of the nose, pinch each eyebrow between the index finger and thumb of each hand. Hold for a few seconds, then release.

❷ Repeating the movement, work outward, away from the nose. When you have covered every part of the brow, repeat again, starting at the bridge of the nose.

circling the temples

Make sure you use enough pressure here to feel the skin move with your fingertips, rather than just making circles on the surface of the skin.

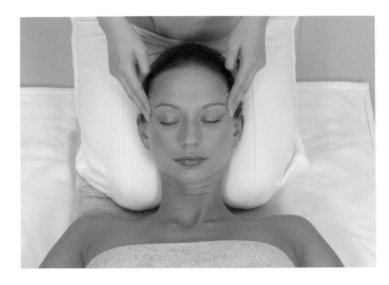

❶ Using your fingertips, locate the very slight hollows of the temples on either side of your partner's eyes.

❷ Very slowly begin to circle your fingertips over and over the spot, working clockwise.

❸ Repeat over the same area, this time circling counterclockwise.

stroking the side of the nose

This technique will help speed up the draining of the sinus cavity. However, only repeat it a few times.

❶ Place your thumbs on either side of the bridge of your partner's nose. Allow your fingers to rest lightly on the outer sides of the face.

❷ Gently glide your thumbs down the nose. As you reach the nostrils, slowly lift your thumbs away. Take them back to the starting position at the bridge of the nose to repeat the stroke.

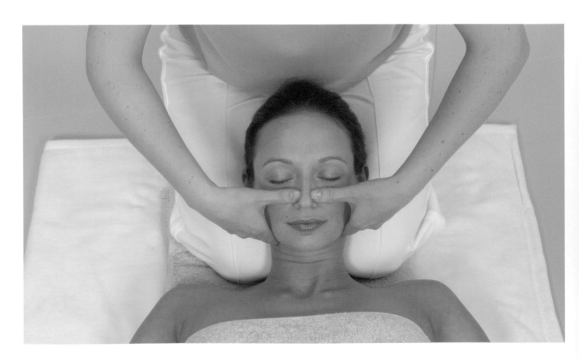

cheek stroke

Remember to keep your fingers in contact with the face at all times during this stroke.

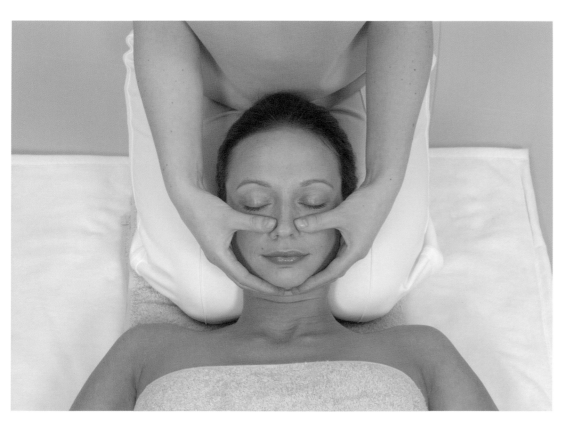

① Place your thumbs on each side of the nose in line with the cheeks. Allow the hands to rest gently on the outsides of the face. Slowly stroke the thumbs out from either side of the nose across each cheek to the outside of the face.

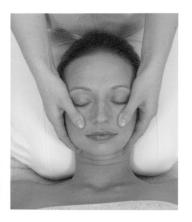
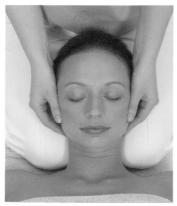
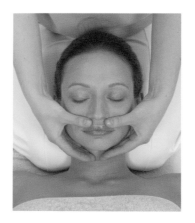
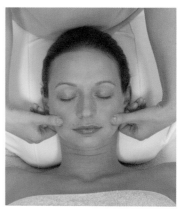

② As your thumbs reach your partner's ears, gently lift them away and return them to the nose area, slightly lower than before. Repeat the movement until you have covered not just the cheekbones, but the entire area of the cheeks.

③ Keeping contact with your fingers, place your thumbs just above the top lip and stroke them out over the lower part of the face. As you reach the jawbone, gently lift your thumbs away and take them back to the starting position to repeat the technique. If desired, repeat below the lower lip.

circular pressure on the cheeks

The point at which the upper and lower jaw meet (the masseter muscle) can be a very tense area; use this technique to help relieve held-in tension.

❶ To find the correct area around which to work, ask your partner to suck their cheeks in.

❷ Place two or three fingertips on each hand on each cheek. Use them to make circular pressure movements all over the area of the cheeks, focusing on areas of tension.

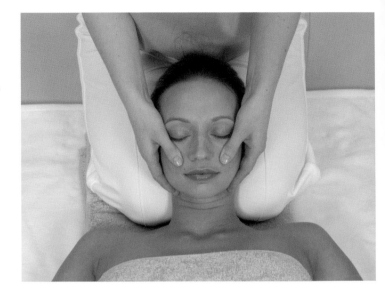

skin rolling

This technique can assist in keeping the skin and muscles of the face toned to deter the tendency toward a double chin.

❶ Place the fingers and thumbs of both hands on the outer side of your partner's jaw, beside the ear. Pinch some skin between your fingers and thumb and very gently roll your curled fingers back toward you, pulling the skin of the jaw while keeping your thumb stationary.

❷ Repeat the movement, gradually working in toward the chin.

❸ Repeat the action in the opposite direction, working back to the ears. This time, gently roll your curled fingers away from you to pull the skin of the jaw toward your stationary thumb.

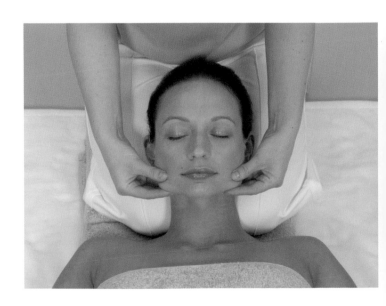

jaw pinch

This sandwiching technique will complement the work of skin rolling to keep the skin elastic and toned.

❶ Make "pincers" with your thumbs and index fingers, then place them on the center of the chin so that the thumbs rest lightly on the top and the index fingers sit slightly under the chin. Gently pinch your thumbs and fingers together, holding the pressure for several seconds, then gently release.

❷ Move your pincers a little way along the jaw, toward the ears, and repeat the movement. Work in the same way along the jawline, out toward the ears.

❸ When you reach the end of the jaw, work your way back toward the center of the chin using the same technique.

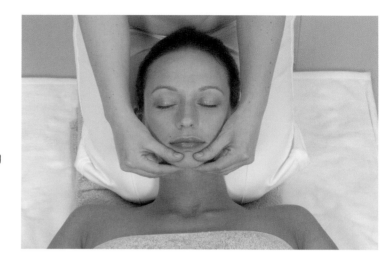

alternate stroking

This stimulates the supply of nutrients to the neck. Keep your hands clear of the throat as you apply this technique.

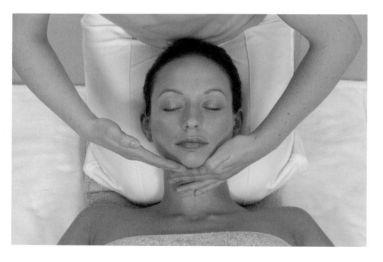

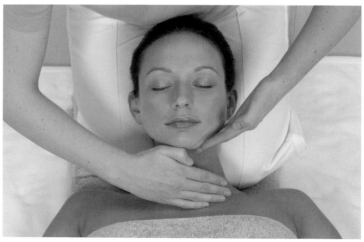

❶ Using the fingertips and palm of one hand, stroke up one side of your partner's neck toward the jawline.

❷ As the first hand reaches the jawline, lift it away and repeat the motion with your other hand on the other side.

❸ Repeat the technique as above, but this time sweeping outward toward the ears on either side of the neck.

stroking the sides of the head

It can feel very reassuring to have the head supported on both sides.

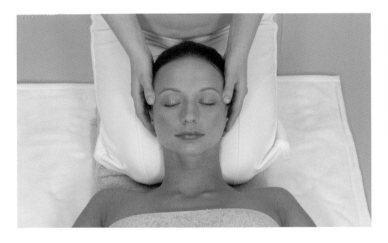

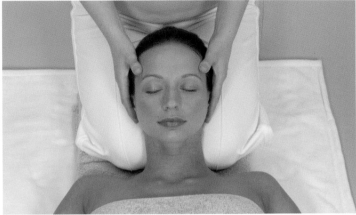

❶ Gently cup the head on either side with the fingers of both hands.

❷ Using the flat part of your thumbs, stroke across the temples and down to the ears.

ear pinch

In Traditional Chinese Medicine, the ear is thought to contain a multitude of pressure points capable of stimulating the whole body.

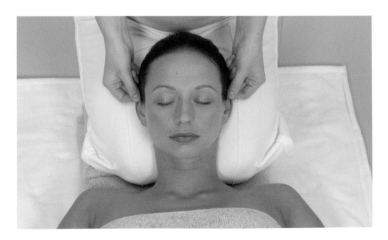

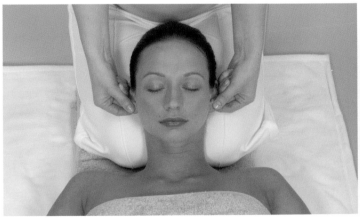

❶ Using your fingertips and thumbs, pinch and release different points all over the top of your partner's ears. This area is said to correspond to the body's extremities.

❷ Continue pinching the fleshy part of the earlobes, working from the bottom to the top. Pinch along the outside of the ear, the part corresponding to the skeletal system.

acupressure points

Applying gentle but firm pressure to acupressure points on the face is thought in Traditional Chinese Medicine (TCM) to help rebalance corresponding areas of the body by enabling qi, life energy, to flow unimpeded.

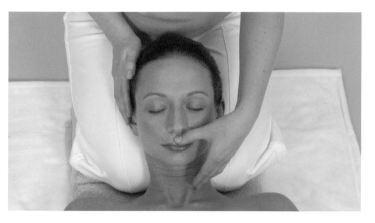

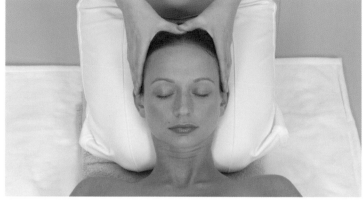

❶ With one finger or thumb, directly apply pressure into the groove below the nose. Hold for several seconds, then release. This is an acupressure point known in TCM as the "governor vessel," which is said to boost concentration and stimulate the senses.

❸ Continue applying pressure up over the center of the head, as far as you can reach on the back of the head.

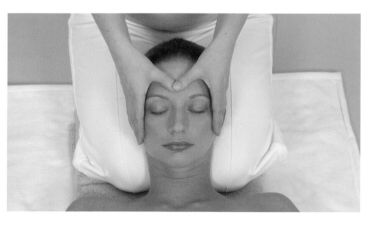

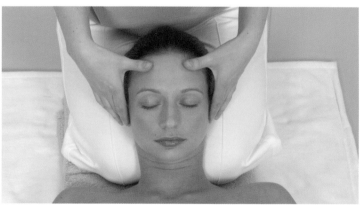

❹ Place your middle fingers on each of your partner's ears and position your thumbs together in the center of the head to locate an acupressure point that is said to improve the general health of the whole body. Lightly press this point, holding for several seconds.

❷ Place your thumb on the center of the forehead just above the bridge of the nose. Place your other thumb on top and apply pressure. Start very gently and increase the pressure slightly as you push in. Hold for several seconds, then release slowly. Repeat two or three times up the center of the forehead toward the hairline.

other techniques for the face

- Raindrops all over, avoiding the eyes (page 51)
- Feathering all over, avoiding the eyes (page 56)

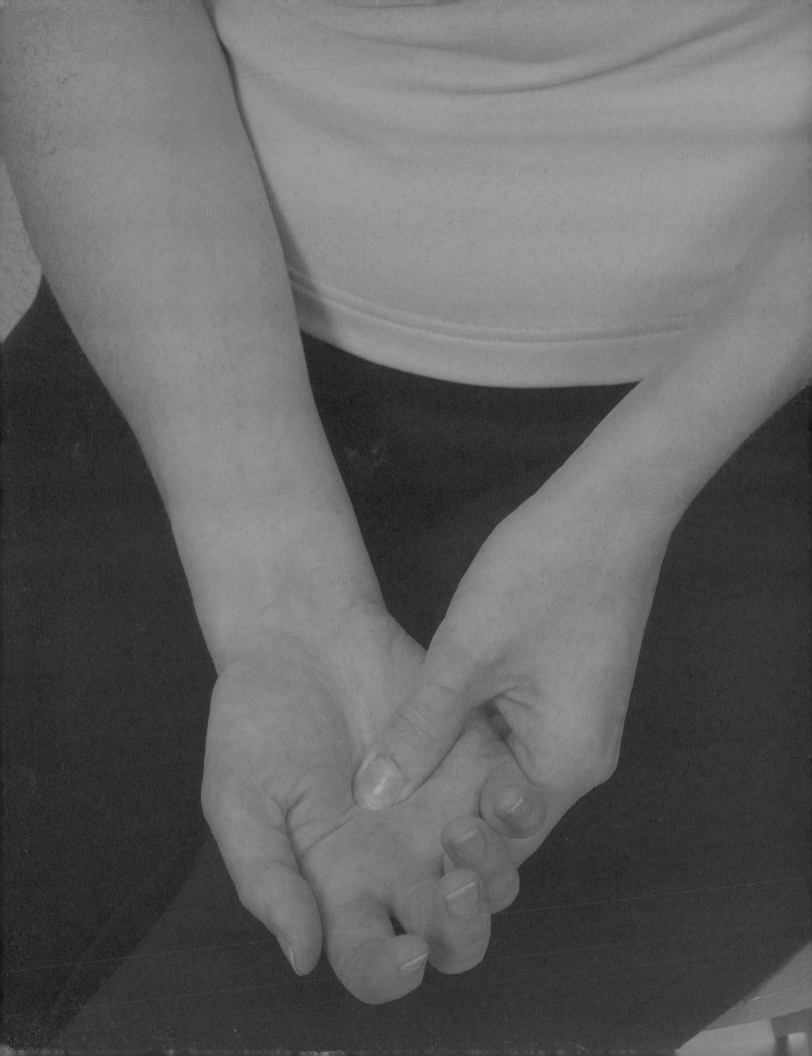

self-massage

While there is nothing like receiving a massage from someone else, it is highly beneficial to be able to apply the techniques to your own body, whether as a pampering treat, at work when you have a stiff neck and shoulders, or after exercising. I always massage my legs after coming off the ski slopes, and then my body is ready for another full day of skiing next day. Use the sequences that follow as a jumping-off point for your own self-massage. You will also find here some essential stretches and postural exercises to keep every part of your body in good shape.

The following pages focus on the legs, neck, and arms. While massaging your own back is a little challenging, the face, feet, chest, and hand sequences from Part 3 can be easily applied to yourself. Complete all the strokes on one leg before massaging the other.

self-massage for the legs

starting position: Sit in a position that is comfortable for you, possibly on a chair (preferably without arms), a stool, or on the side of a bed. Apply oil all over the leg using gentle, sweeping strokes.

effleurage for the legs

Make the pulling up of this technique much firmer than the stroking down.

❶ With fingers and thumbs together and one hand above the other, cup your hands around the front of your thigh and stroke them down the entire length of your leg, gliding very lightly over the knee.

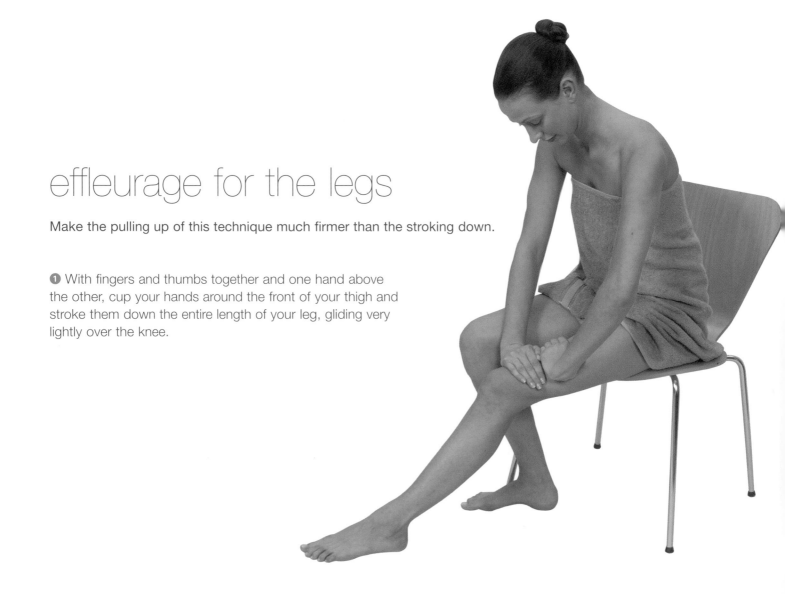

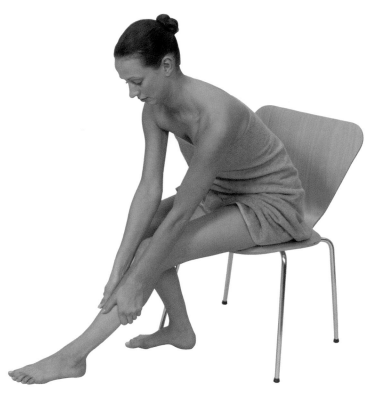

② As your hands approach the ankle, sweep your fingers outward and pull up the outside of the leg, back to your starting point on the thigh, ready to repeat the whole movement. If desired, take your hands around the back of the leg on the return stroke so that you massage the entire limb.

open-handed kneading on the calf

Lift one leg and rest the foot on the knee of the other leg.

❶ Perform the open-handed kneading technique shown on page 64 on your calf. Work first on the back of the calf.

❷ Repeat the technique more lightly over the front of the lower leg. Rock from side to side to help incorporate body weight into the movement.

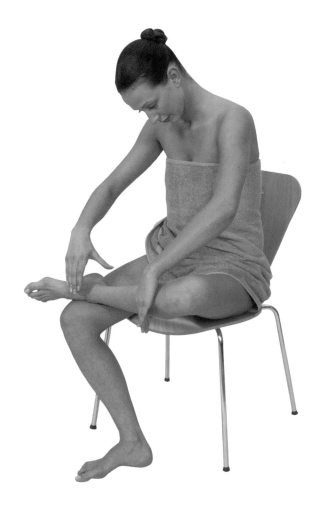

open-handed kneading on the thigh

Bend the knee and support the foot on whatever you are sitting on.

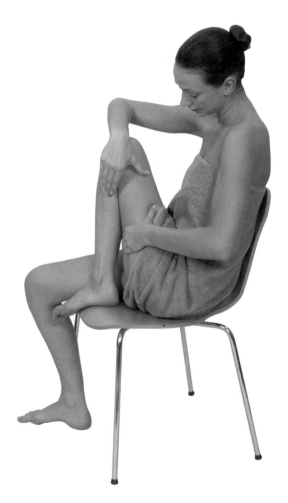

❶ Perform the open-handed kneading technique described on page 64, working this time on the top of the thigh.

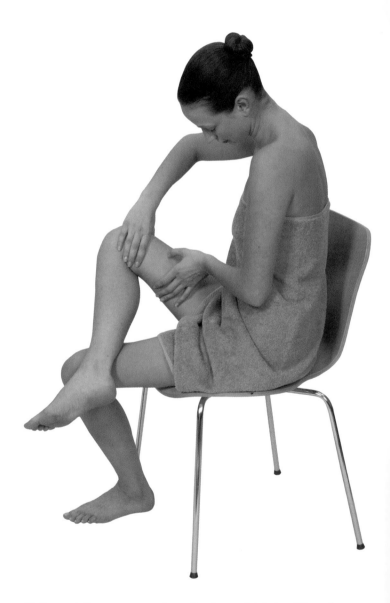

❷ Repeat the movement on the inner thigh by tilting the knee outward, and then on the outside of the thigh by tilting the knee inward.

alternate kneading sitting on a chair

Sitting in the same position, now alternate your hands.

❶ Place one hand on some muscle of the thigh and grasp the muscle between the fingers and the thumb. Pull the muscle with the fingers toward your stationary thumb, allowing the muscle to gradually escape from your grasp. As this hand is about to finish, repeat with the other hand.

❷ Repeat the stroke wherever you find tightness and tension. Use your body weight to ensure that your thumbs are not doing all the work.

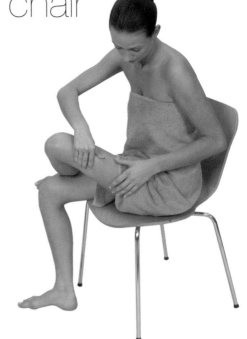

circular pressure on the thigh and calf

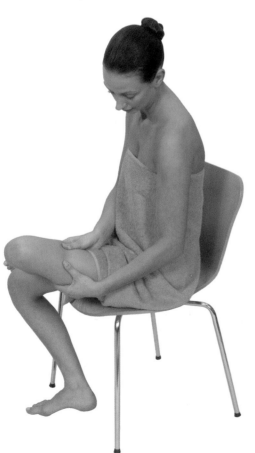

Finish your self-massage for the leg with stress-relieving deep pressure work.

❶ Use the pad of one or both thumbs to make slow, deep circular strokes all over the thigh. Pay special attention to particular areas of tension and tightness.

❷ Repeat the movement on the back of the calf.

❸ Soothe the thigh and calf by repeating the long, gentle effleurage routine on page 142 to finish work on this leg. Repeat all the strokes on the other leg.

self-massage for the neck and shoulders

When you find yourself sitting hunched in front of the computer monitor, take five minutes every now and then to relieve the tension in your neck and shoulders with the following strokes.

starting position: Sit comfortably on a chair. No oil is required for this massage.

do-in

Sometimes vigorous stimulation is required to encourage the muscle to release its tension. Try this Japanese method.

stroking

Prepare the muscle for deeper work with long, sweeping strokes.

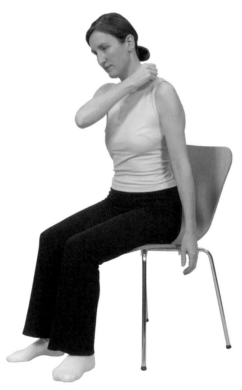

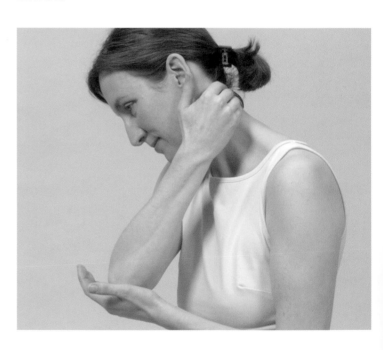

❶ Tilt your head to one side and place one hand (fingers and thumbs together) on the back of the other shoulder, supporting the weight of your arm at the elbow with your other hand.

❶ Make a fist with your supported hand and vigorously pound the muscles of the shoulder all over.

❷ Repeat the technique on your other shoulder.

❷ Stroke up and down the side of the neck and back of the shoulder from your hairline. Lift the hand away and return it to your starting position to repeat the stroke.

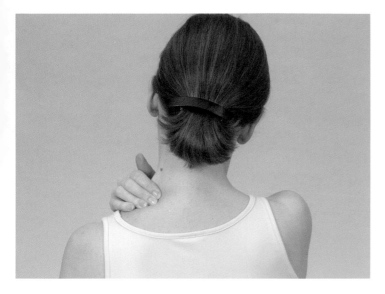

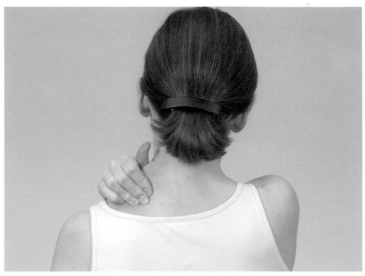

circular pressure

Now work more deeply on areas of tightness.

❶ Maintaining the same arm position, make deep, slow, circular strokes with the fingertips all over the back of your opposite shoulder, wherever the muscles feel tense and tight.

❷ Repeat the stroke over the side of the neck.

squeeze and hold

This breaks down held-in tension even further.

Again in the same supported arm position, grasp the muscle on the top of the shoulder between the heel of your hand and your fingertips. Squeeze the muscle and hold for 8–10 seconds before gently releasing.

pressure on the back of the neck

Never work directly on the spine itself.

❶ Place the fingertips of both hands on the back of your neck, positioned on either side of the spine at the base of the neck.

❷ Make deep, slow, circular strokes all over this area and into the base of the skull.

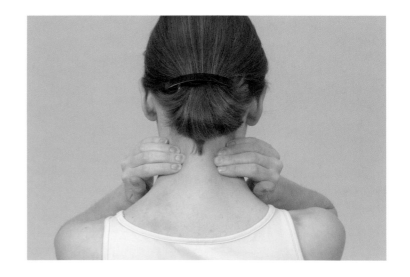

self-massage for the arms

Tension in the arms can cause the shoulders and neck to ache, so if your day involves working at the computer, carrying or lifting, or other repetitive tasks, make sure to ease the arm muscles with these simple self-massage strokes. Perform all the techniques on one arm before turning your attention to the other one.

starting position: Sit in a comfortable position with your arm resting on your lap. Apply oil all over the arm using gentle sweeping strokes.

effleurage for the arm

Make the upward stroke much firmer than the downward stroke.

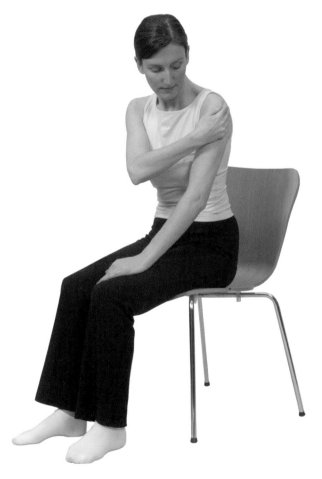

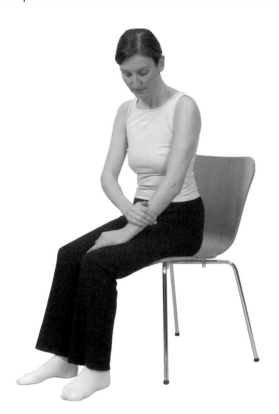

❶ Keeping the fingers and thumbs of your working hand together, cup the hand around the top of your opposite wrist and stroke up the entire length of the arm, gliding very lightly over the elbow.

❷ Stroke your hand firmly around the shoulder joint, then glide gently down the outside of the arm, ready to repeat the whole movement.

❸ If desired, repeat the stroke along the length of the inner arm, from the inside of the wrist to beneath the underarm.

circular pressure around the arm

Lay your forearm across your lap with the palm facing upward.

1 Using the pad of the thumb of your working hand, make slow, deep, circular strokes all over the inside of your relaxed arm. Work into particular areas of tension and tightness.

2 Soothe the entire area with gentle effleurage, as before.

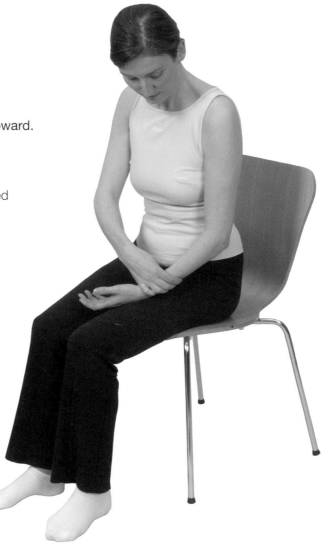

circular pressure on the palm

Now place your hand palm upward, resting on one thigh.

1 Using the pad of the thumb of your working hand, make slow, deep circular strokes all over the palm and fingers of your relaxed hand.

2 Soothe the whole hand with gentle effleurage strokes, as before.

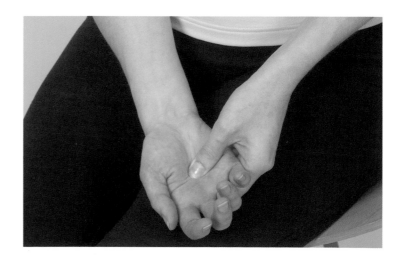

self-help stretches

The techniques that follow are invaluable for anyone with a busy lifestyle, helping to rebalance a body that has become misaligned by tight muscles. After giving a massage, you can use these exercises to realign your posture, which can become strained as a result of long periods spent sitting.

back rest

Through everyday overuse and misuse, the muscles in the back become overtight and out of balance. It is important to regularly allow these muscles to rest. Try this simple but effective exercise.

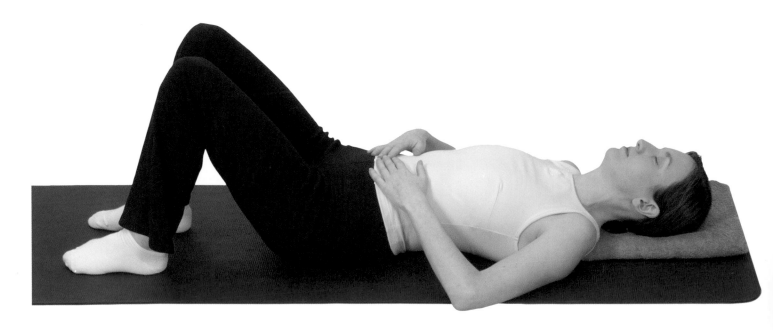

❶ Lie on your back on the floor with knees bent and feet flat on the ground. You could place a folded towel beneath your head to keep the spine in alignment.

❷ Rest your hands by your sides or on your stomach, and relax for 10–15 minutes.

rhomboid stretch

The muscles between the shoulder blades, known as the rhomboids, can get very tight and tense, creating aches in the upper back. Use this stretch during the day to ease them out.

❶ Interlock the fingers of both hands and turn the backs of the hands in toward you.

❷ Relax your head toward your chest and push your arms away from you until you feel a pull in the upper back. This should not be painful, but may be mildly uncomfortable. Hold the stretch for 10–15 seconds, then slowly release. Keep breathing as you stretch.

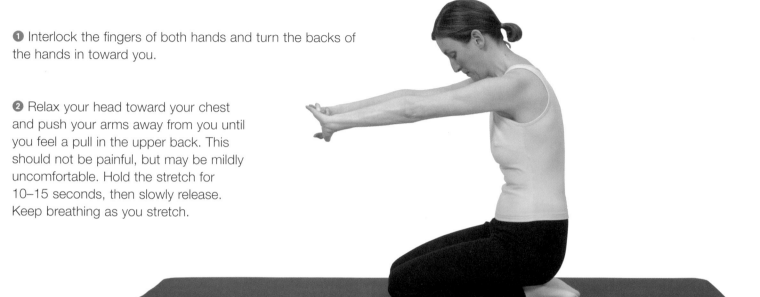

lying stretch

During the course of the day, gravity causes the disks between the vertebrae of the spine to become compressed; we may even shrink by one or two inches. Let this stretch help elongate the spine.

❶ Lie on your back and stretch your arms behind your head, pointing your toes at the same time, as if trying to make yourself as tall as possible.

❷ Hold for 10–15 seconds, breathing slowly and deeply, before relaxing.

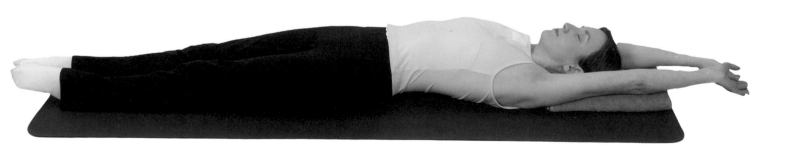

calf stretch

Use this to counter the stress of wearing high heels.

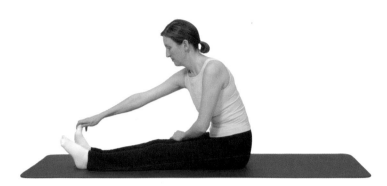

❶ Sit on the floor with legs outstretched in front of you. Lean forward over one leg and take hold of your toes.

❷ Pull the toes slowly toward you until you feel a stretch in the back of the calf. Hold for 10–20 seconds, then slowly release. Repeat on the other leg.

hamstring stretch

Men especially suffer from tense, short hamstrings and benefit from increased flexibility at the back of the thighs.

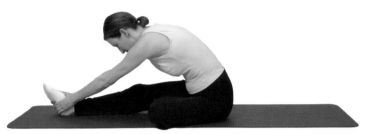

❶ Maintaining the position of the calf stretch, release your toes and relax your ankle. Pull one foot up to rest against the opposite inner thigh, allowing the knee to fall away from the body.

❷ Pivot forward from the hips with a straight back to lean over the legs until you feel a pull at the back of the thigh. Hold the stretch for 10–20 seconds, then slowly release.

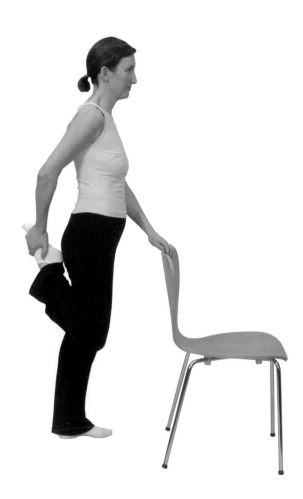

quadriceps stretch

Sitting for long periods causes this important muscle to shorten, which adversely affects the posture.

❶ Stand holding the back of a chair or a wall for support. Take the foot of one leg back toward your buttocks.

❷ With your hand, slowly pull your foot as close as possible toward your buttocks without causing discomfort. Tilt your hips forward to increase the stretch, keeping the knees together. You should feel a pull on the front of the thigh. Hold for 10–20 seconds, then slowly release. Repeat on the other leg.

leg relaxation

People who spend all day on their feet often end up with tired, aching, even swollen legs and feet. This position counters such problems in a very relaxing way.

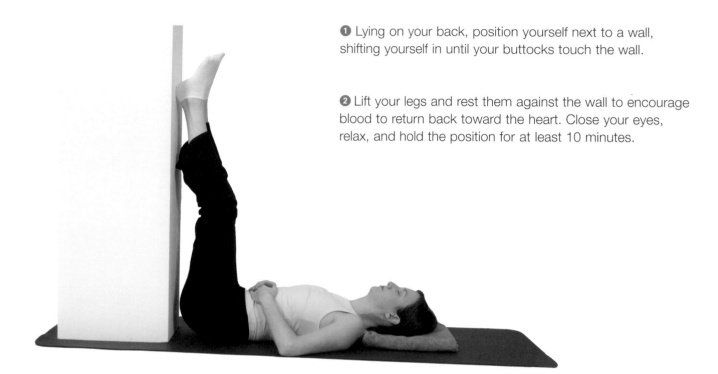

❶ Lying on your back, position yourself next to a wall, shifting yourself in until your buttocks touch the wall.

❷ Lift your legs and rest them against the wall to encourage blood to return back toward the heart. Close your eyes, relax, and hold the position for at least 10 minutes.

neck stretch

There is a large, triangular muscle called the trapezius that spans the shoulders, attaching to the shoulder blade and going up the side of the neck to the skull. As tension seems to reside here, it helps to stretch the neck muscles.

❶ Tilt your head, taking one ear toward its shoulder. Stop when you feel a slight pull in the opposite side of the neck.

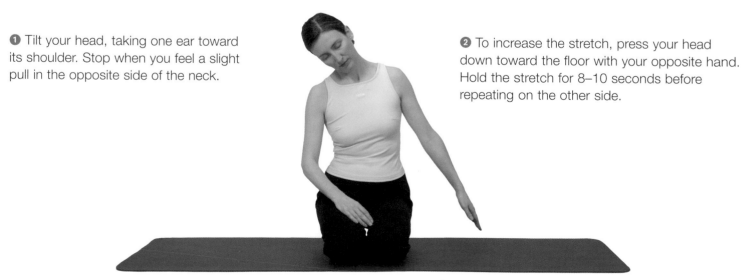

❷ To increase the stretch, press your head down toward the floor with your opposite hand. Hold the stretch for 8–10 seconds before repeating on the other side.

neck and back stretch

This twist rejuvenates the length of the spine by encouraging space to develop between each vertebra.

❶ Sit on the floor with legs extended in front of you. Cross your right leg over your left leg and place your right foot flat on the floor beside your left knee.

❷ Rotating your body clockwise, place your right hand on the floor as close to your right buttock as possible. Extend your left arm, and placing it across your left knee, use it as a lever to push you even further to the right. Turn your head to look as far behind you as possible. Hold for 10 seconds or longer.

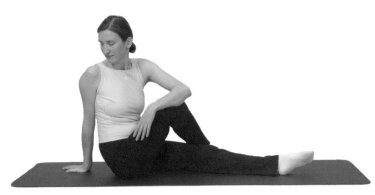

triceps stretch

Perform this stretch from a sitting or standing position.

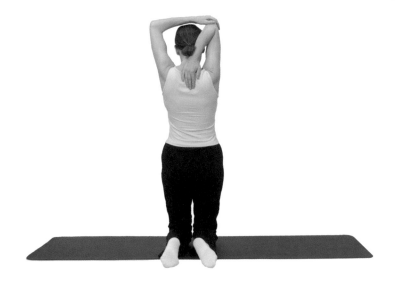

❶ Take one arm over and behind your head, resting the palm between your shoulder blades.

❷ Place your other hand on the elbow of the bent arm and press down gently until you feel a slight pull along the outside of the upper bent arm. Hold for 8–10 seconds, and then come out of the stretch slowly. Repeat on the other arm.

pectoral stretch

Remember to breathe in and out deeply as you hold this position to increase the stretch.

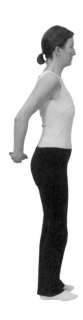

❶ Standing up straight, clasp your hands behind your back by interlocking your fingers.

❷ Keeping your arms slightly bent, lift them up and back until you feel a stretch in the pectoral muscles of the chest. Hold the stretch for 8–10 seconds before relaxing.

finger stretch

This exercise encourages flexibility in the fingers and helps them relax after giving a massage.

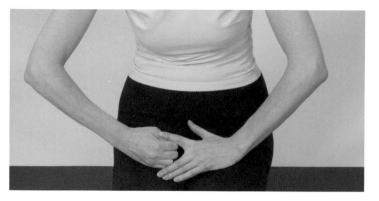

❶ Make a fist with one hand and wedge it between two fingers of the other hand for several seconds to stretch the hand out.

❷ Repeat between all the fingers several times. Repeat on the other hand.

foot relaxation

Relax your feet in a bowl of warm water with some bath salts, close your eyes, and consciously relax every inch of your body. Invest in a foot roller to stimulate, exercise, and relax all the muscles of the foot. A roller also stimulates pressure points found in the feet that are treated in reflexology to rebalance every part of the body.

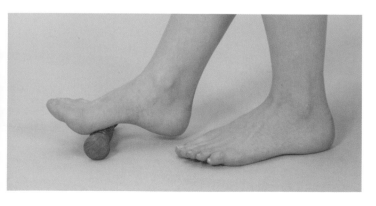

wrist strengthener

If you suffer from weak wrists, it is possible to strengthen them with the following exercise.

❶ Take a weight, such as a can of soup, and hold it with your palm facing down and your forearm resting on the edge of a surface, such as the arm of a chair or a table edge.

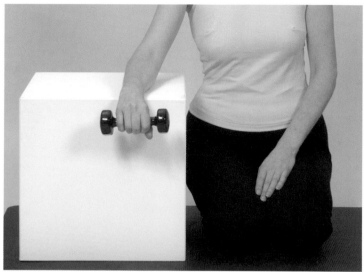

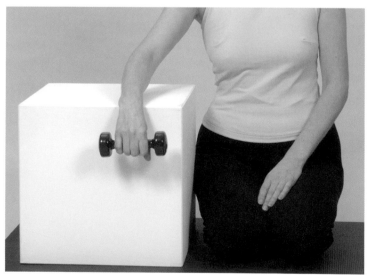

❷ Lift and lower your hand slowly and with control by flexing the wrist. Repeat with the other arm.

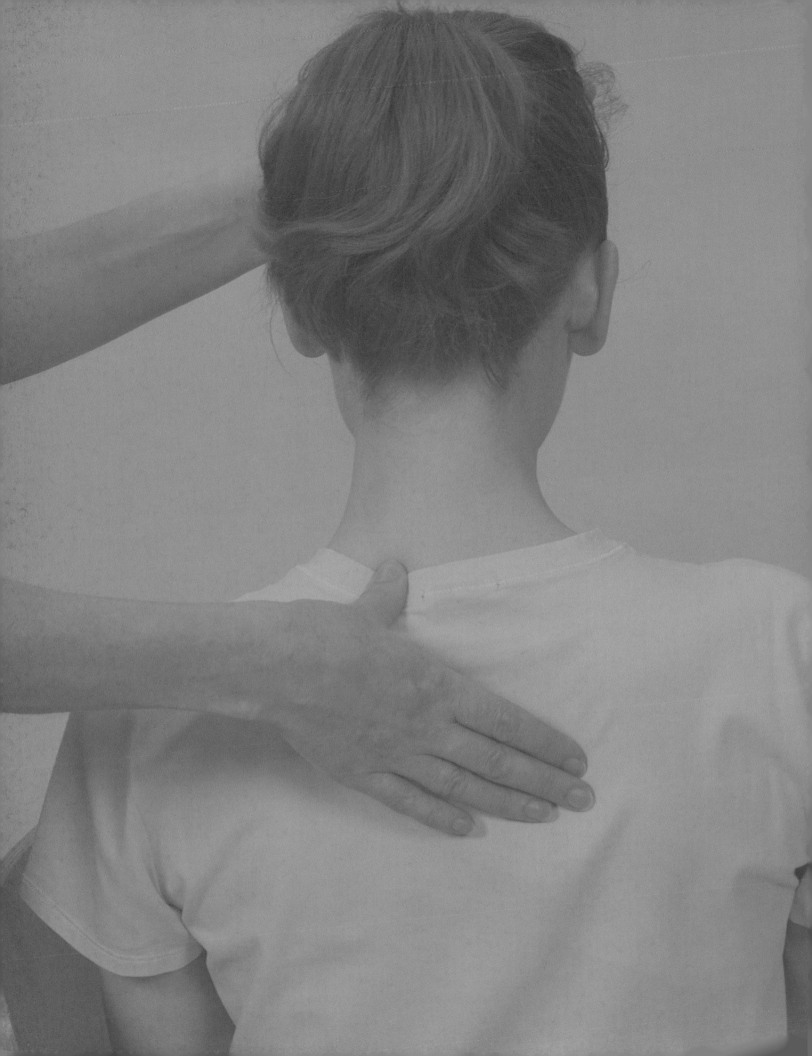

massage programs

Here are effective ways to bring massage into every part of your life: routines for the bedroom and the boardroom, strokes to relieve the symptoms of ill health, and sequences for every member of the family to follow at any time of life, from childhood to our later years.

sensual massage

For thousands of years, touch and massage have played a part in lovemaking, and rightly so. Touch allows you to get to know your partner—to discover sensitivities and explore what pleases most. Massage conveys a strong sense of loving and forges a deep level of trust and openness. In today's fast-track society, massage in the bedroom brings back the sacredness of the sexual act. To share ecstasy with your partner and make lovemaking sublime is truly an act of love.

how to massage

All the techniques in this book are perfect for use in the bedroom between two lovers as an exquisite part of lovemaking. Given with the thought and intention to be sensual and performed delicately, provocatively, and with lingering fingers, all the techniques heighten arousal while enhancing and prolonging the pleasure of sexual intimacy. Be creative and playful, exploring gentle strokes and techniques on sensitive and erogenous areas of the body.

Ensure you have your partner's agreement before embarking on a sensual massage in order to make sure he or she doesn't expect a relaxation massage.

heightening sensitivity

When giving a sensual massage, work with your fingertips and focus on sensitive areas of the body rather than on muscles: try the inside of the knees and elbows, the nape of the neck, the ears, the fingers, the toes, the abdomen, the hair. Your partner's body will purr in appreciation. Listed below are some of the massage techniques that you can bring to a sensual massage.

a light finger stroked down the thigh

Keeping the pressure light, stroke your fingertips down your partner's thigh. Take the time to appreciate the texture, appearance, and warmth of the skin. Slow movements are best, lingering in one place for a while before tantalizingly and slowly moving on.

stroking with the hair

Sensual massage is an open invitation to imaginative massage. If you have long hair, try stroking your hair across your partner's skin. It will be featherlight and watching your partner's reaction is a good way of establishing a new closeness between the two of you.

teasing the hair

Gentle pulling of the hair not only enlivens your partner's scalp and hair follicles, it is also a good way of easing out tension from the head and neck, helping your partner to relax even deeper into the massage. You can continue this relaxation by moving down the neck to gently knead the shoulder and neck muscles.

blowing on the skin

The intimacy and trust shared by a couple allows them to experiment with massage. Try blowing on your partner's skin to bring a new sensation to the massage, allowing your partner to really appreciate the different sensations that can be transmitted through the skin.

the right environment for a sensual massage

Sensual massage is all about mood. So try to choose a time of day when you and your partner will both be relaxed and open, with no tasks or appointments to worry about. Make sure that the room you are in is warm and private. It may be a good idea to clear away any clutter, as these could act as unwelcome reminders of the outside world and commitments. Choose suitable mood music, light candles, and burn aromatherapy oils. All of this will help you both establish and enjoy the intimacy of the massage.

have fun

Remember that you are with someone you love and trust. Don't take your sensual massage too seriously and you'll be able to relax even if you feel shy. This is a time for you and your partner to enjoy yourselves and each other, so even if you end up laughing, you are still enjoying the benefits of a good massage experience!

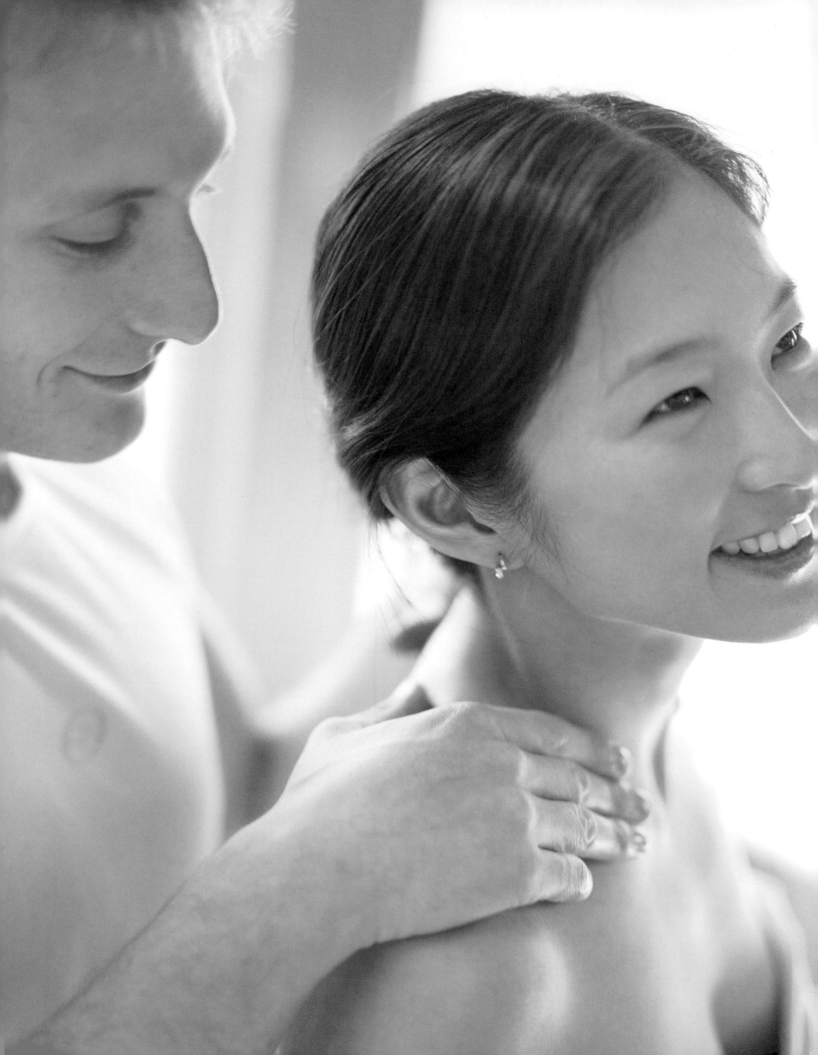

massage for pregnancy

The trend in the West for moving back to more natural and simple ways of being is never so true as in pregnancy and childbirth. Massage has a vital role to play in this pilgrimage. Traditional maternity care included massage, and it is encouraging to see it once again taking up this important place. Massage during pregnancy, when performed by a partner, can enhance and develop the bond you both have with your unborn child. It also brings you closer as a couple and provides a wonderful way of remaining intimate if lovemaking becomes less frequent. It helps your partner feel much more involved in the pregnancy and will encourage him or her to be active in the birth and child-raising.

the benefits of massage

Massage can help a woman accept the changes in her body as pregnancy progresses, enhancing self-esteem and relieving tension. It is also very effective at easing many of the side effects of being pregnant. Massage in pregnancy can ease backaches, leg cramps, headaches, and swollen ankles and feet. It can help keep blood pressure in check by aiding circulation and encouraging deep breathing, and can relieve digestive disorders. Massage and oils can help the skin maintain its elasticity. It can also improve circulation to the fetus, assisting in its healthy development.

cautions

There are only a few contraindications to massage in pregnancy, but you should always refer to the safety guidelines on page 38:

- Undiagnosed vaginal bleeding: find out the cause before giving massage.
- Preeclampsia: although as long as this is being monitored, massage can be beneficial.
- Abdominal pain: obtain permission from your partner's midwife or doctor before giving massage.

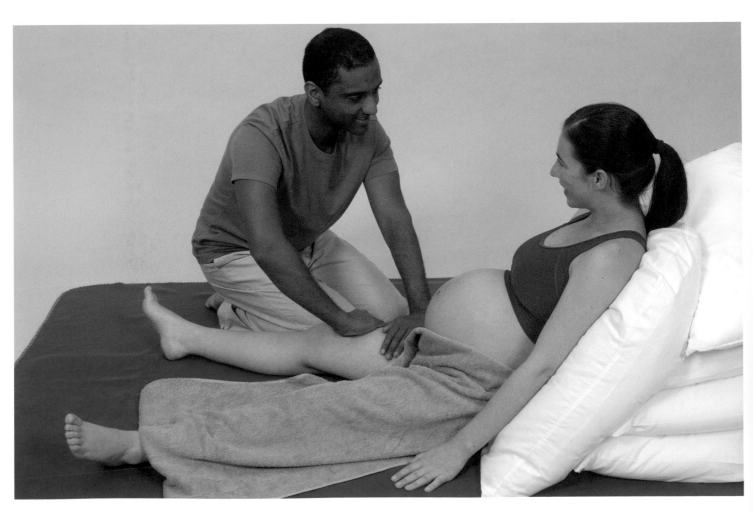

how to massage

Many of the techniques in this book can be used to massage a pregnant woman, but avoid any massage on the abdomen except light effleurage and holding techniques. Also avoid pressure work around the lower back, ankles, and shoulders, as these contain pressure points that can stimulate contractions.

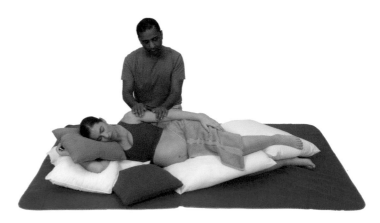

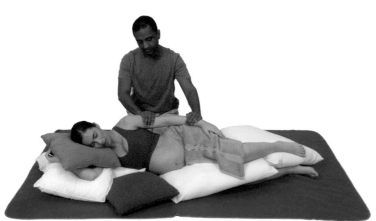

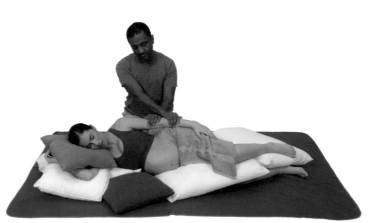

positioning a pregnant woman

First trimester: It is acceptable for an expectant mother to lie on her stomach during the first trimester (up to twelve weeks), provided she feels comfortable.

Second trimester: Give massage with the expectant mother lying on her side. Use cushions to make her comfortable: under her neck, upper leg (for the lower leg to rest on), maybe under the bump, and

the arms—whatever seems most comfortable. It makes sense, if the mother is comfortable, to perform massage first on one side and then the other.

Third trimester: The mother may feel restless and need to move around a little more. You can begin to include work with the mother in an all-fours position both to give her a break and to assist the baby into a good position for labor.

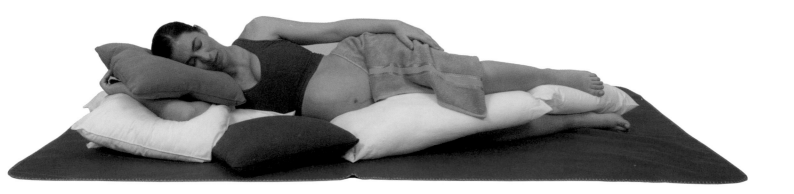

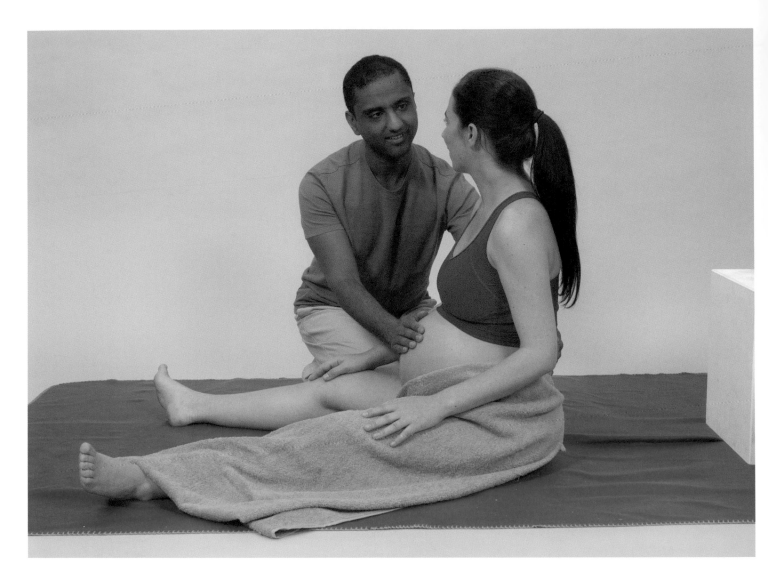

connecting with the baby

For the pregnant woman's partner to feel like an important part of the
pregnancy and to feel connected to his or her child before it is born,
there are some simple techniques that can be used regularly to create
a powerful bond.

1. Place one hand above the navel and the other hand beneath the
spine, directly opposite the other. Imagine energy bouncing from one
hand to the other.

2. Spend a couple of minutes on the technique until you start to feel a
"spreading" sensation between your hands. You may even find that
you are able to make a connection with the baby. Remove your hands
slowly.

3. Imagine tuning in to the baby in the womb through the warmth of
your hands and the energy of your thoughts.

4. Breathe in time with your partner as you open your hearts to
sending love, safety, and warmth to your developing child.

the use of transitions for working around the body

When working on the expectant mother's side, it is harder to do long,
sweeping effleurage strokes. However, you can make effective
transitions simply by placing your hand on one area and then moving
to another. This gives a sense of continuity and flow. You can also use
simple, passive movements by holding parts of the body. These are
effective for relaxing limbs and joints and improving blood flow.

abdominal work

1. Place one hand on the abdomen and one hand on the lower back.

2. With the hand on the abdomen, apply pressure by drawing the two
hands together as your partner breathes out. Make sure the pressure
feels comfortable and appropriate. Tune in to the baby in the womb,
as well as the mother. Firm pressure, if applied sensitively and
gradually, is usually preferable to a pressure that is too light. As your
partner breathes in, release some of the pressure but keep contact.
Repeat this a few times.

3. Continue to work in this way around the abdomen in a clockwise direction. You can work around a second time with a closer or wider circle away from the navel.

nausea

For nausea, you can also press on an acupressure point found two thumb widths down from the wrist crease in the center of arm. Use as often and as long as feels comfortable.

massage in labor

During labor, every woman's needs are very different and some may not want massage at all. If a woman is open to massage during labor, the main areas that need to be worked are the sacrum and lower back, the abdomen, the neck and shoulders, the legs, the arms, and the feet. Women tend to respond better to holding techniques— simply holding a part of the body firmly during contractions—as there is so much going on during labor. However, between contractions, they may like effleurage techniques.

the sacrum

Massage of the lower back and sacrum can be beneficial—firm, slow effleurage can be pain-relieving. It is an extremely helpful area to apply pressure to, as it can often feel pained in labor. It also relaxes the whole pelvis, can provide pain relief, and allows labor to progress. Between contractions, gentle stroking or lighter general pressure can help with relaxation.

general relaxation of the sacrum

Two-handed technique:

1. Place one hand on top of the other. The fingers of the lower hand point up the spine, the upper hand is at 90 degrees to the lower hand. Lean into the two hands, applying pressure on the partner's out breath. Work for at least three-quarters of the out breaths on one area and gradually work down the sacrum, including over the coccyx.

2. Kneading and stroking of the buttocks is appropriate at this stage.

the abdomen

Touch here may help with pain relief, and it can also help connect the parents with the baby. Use gentle, clockwise stroking or gentle pressure. You can use effleurage techniques to stroke from front to back and link with massaging the sacrum.

pain relief in labor

The following shiatsu pressure points are very effective in offering pain relief during labor. They are also useful in prolonged labor if contractions are ineffectual or if there are any difficulties in getting labor started.

These points should not be stimulated before labor begins, as they could lead to miscarriage. Those who aren't pregnant also find some of these points helpful for pain relief.

- "Spleen 6" Place the tip of your little finger on top of the ankle bone of the opposite leg, fingers pointing to the front of the leg. This point lies beneath the second joint of the forefinger, under the shin.
- "Liver 3" On top of the foot between the first and second toes, i.e., between the first and second metatarsal bones.
- "Gallbladder 21" In the hollow on top of the shoulder, straight up from the nipple when you are standing. It is in the highest point of the shoulder. This can be incorporated in a shoulder massage, which is relaxing for the woman in labor. It releases tension in the shoulder, neck, and jaw. It can also be of help with poor lactation.
- "Large intestine 4" Between the thumb and index finger on the back of the hand. To locate, have the thumb and index finger closed and the point is at the highest spot of the muscle.

baby massage

In my travels around the world, particularly in Asian countries, I have often watched mothers sitting in the shade, massaging their babies in their laps. Watching this natural, effortless, and loving gift that is so obviously a pleasure for both mother and baby really brings home what we in the West are missing out on. We have much to relearn and remember to become attuned to a more natural, peaceful, tactile, and loving way of being. The sequences that follow offer a taste of baby massage, but for the best results find a class where you will have the support and guidance of a trained instructor as you learn the techniques and enjoy the companionship of other new parents and time away from daily tasks at home.

the benefits of baby massage

Babies not only reap the same benefits from massage as adults (page 16), they gain advantages from loving touch that are absolutely fundamental to an infant's well-being. Insufficient loving touch for all of us, but particularly babies, can lead to withdrawal, depression, and lack of appetite. Scientists now acknowledge that if babies do not receive adequate loving, tactile stimulation, they can be adversely affected psychologically.

Massage encourages mothers and fathers to make eye contact with and smile, stroke, and talk to a baby, all of which are crucial in developing a loving parent-child bond. Massage opens up the communication between parent and baby, and develops the adult's ability to understand how a baby communicates with his or her body.

specific benefits

- Stimulates the functioning and development of all the baby's body systems
- Provides relief from common complaints, such as teething, colic, and constipation
- Enhances relaxation: studies show reduced stress levels in massaged infants, even premature babies.

benefits for parents

- Improves self-confidence
- Promotes bonding
- Enhances the ability to read a baby's body language and nonverbal cues
- Produces relaxing hormones during the massage

when to massage

You can massage your baby every day or however often your lifestyle allows. Routine brings a sense of security to babies, so choose a time of day suitable for both your baby and yourself. It is important to treat children with the utmost respect and to gain their permission before giving a massage. Even the youngest baby can indicate through body language whether he or she is feeling comfortable or not. Teaching children that they can communicate whether they wish to be touched or not will serve them well in later life.

Observe your baby; when he or she is ready for massage, his or her movements will be quiet and slow, and he or she will make eye contact and show an obvious readiness to interact.

You can massage your baby as soon as he or she feels comfortable with it. Many newborns feel vulnerable being naked and exposed, so swaddle him or her in a towel, have him or her on your lap, and massage a small part of the body at a time. You can continue to massage your babies and children all through their childhoods. As babies get older and start to crawl, you can make it a game or give the massage just before bedtime or after a bath.

when not to massage

Research shows that the best time for a baby to receive massage is when he or she is in a quiet, alert state. Do not massage your baby while he or she is asleep, when tired or hungry, or just after a feeding. If your baby cries during the massage, accept that he or she has had enough or is not in the mood, and offer a cuddle instead.

how to massage

Use a light, pure, organic vegetable oil, such as sunflower, to massage your baby; avoid those containing additives or essential oils. Perform the techniques with care and with a firm, even pressure to avoid tickling and irritating your infant. Most importantly, focus on the quality of your connection rather than the techniques. As long as you work caringly and lovingly, there really is no right or wrong way to massage a baby.

beginning the massage

In my baby massage classes, it is always a pleasure to start with a guided relaxation for the parents and to find that, as we all relax, the babies more often than not relax and become quiet too. I believe that babies come into the world with wonderful perceptions and intuitions and can pick up on our feelings and emotions and often mirror them. Babies also have their own emotions; massage and quality touch give them the safe environment and self-esteem to express them. Start your baby massage by lying on the floor next to your baby. Close your eyes, relax your limbs, and focus on your breathing, letting it become deeper and slower. Watch how your baby relaxes too.

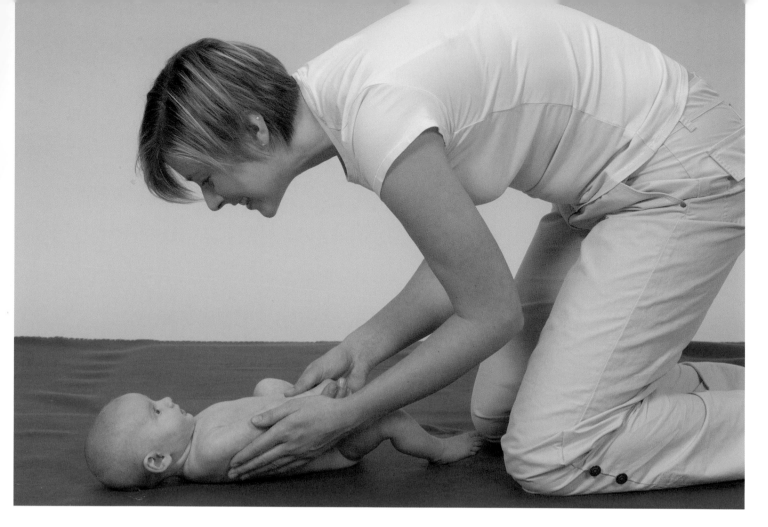

swishing oil

Make sure your baby is open and willing to receive a massage. This sets the standard for a respectful and supportive relationship as your child grows. Communicate your intention to give a massage by swishing some oil between the hands and asking the baby if he or she would like a massage. Babies quickly learn to associate these sounds and actions with massage, and you will soon be able to pick up on body language and other cues telling you yes or no. Yes cues include open body language and a willingness to maintain eye contact. Turning the head and pulling away are signs that an infant is not in the mood.

stroking techniques

You can massage your baby all over his or her body with firm stroking techniques, as described below.

stroking the legs

Support your baby's foot with one hand. Cup the fingers of your working hand around the limb, and using careful but firm pressure, glide your hand up the length of the leg. Sweep down the outside of the limb, ready to repeat the stroke.

circular pressure

Still supporting the foot, circle the thumb of the other hand slowly into the muscular areas of the leg, such as the back of the calf and thigh.

oiling the feet

With firm contact, massage oil into the top and sole of one foot, then the other.

stroking the tummy

Carefully place your hand on your infant's abdomen and rest it there for a while. With a firm, sweeping motion, stroke around the navel in a clockwise direction to aid digestion.

stroking the back

Place one hand on either side of the spine. Stroke up the length of the back, over the shoulders, and down the outside of the body to the buttocks, ready to start again.

arm massage

Repeat the techniques you used on the legs and feet on the arms and hands.

face massage

Making eye contact, place your thumbs gently on the center of your baby's forehead, and stroke them out across the forehead. Stroke down across the cheeks and out across the top lip.

family massage

The ancient Hawaiian massage tradition of lomi lomi offers a wonderfully simple yet powerful sequence that can be performed over clothes. It is a fun activity that is particularly appropriate for families, enabling a loving, physical connection to be maintained as children grow up. The sequence presented here is taught by Serge Kahili King, who learned it from the Kahili family of Kauai, an island of Hawaii.

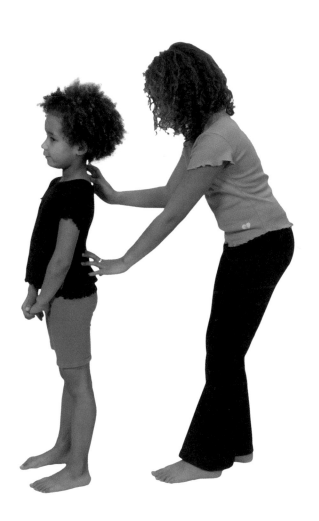

1. kahi ahi fire or glowing heat
Using the fingertips and starting at the front of the scalp, firmly but gently rake the skin downward over all the surfaces of the body except the face, chest, and abdomen. Imagine you are raking coals from a fire.

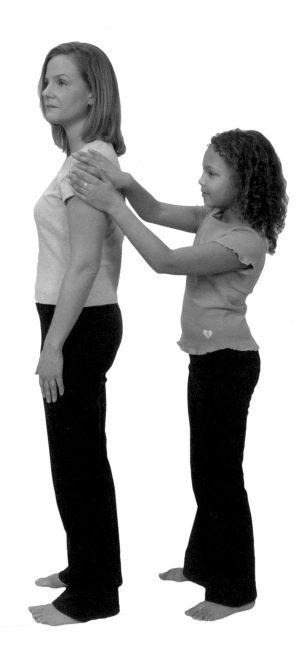

2. kahi wai flowing water
Starting at the head, caress the entire body as if your hands were made of water, rippling, eddying and flowing, circling around joints and points of tension.

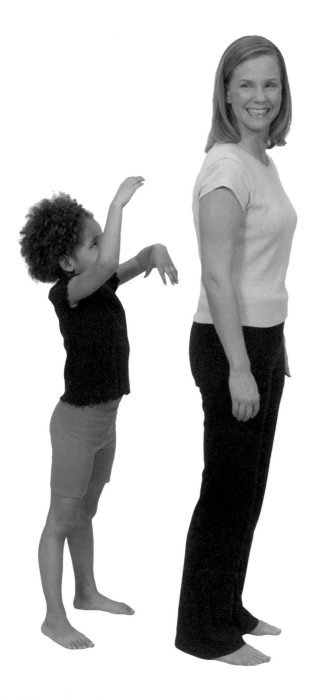

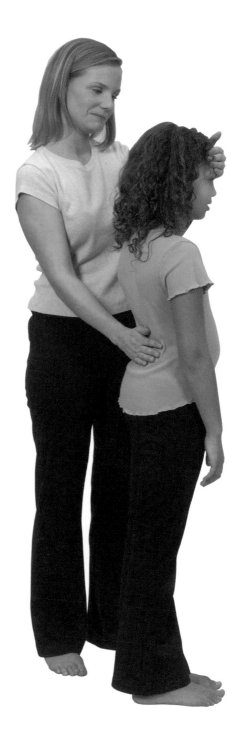

3. kahi makani moving wind

Holding your hands over the body about 4–6 inches above the skin, briskly flap your hands from the wrist to waft currents of air over the body. Imagine this action is loosening or smoothing any areas of resistance as if you were actually making physical changes to the body.

4. kahi pohaku radiant crystal energy

Place one hand at the site of a healthy joint or organ, at the navel, on a known acupressure point, or on a chakra (at the pelvis, abdomen, solar plexus, heart, throat, third eye area, and crown of the head). Place the other hand on a site of tension or pain. Breathe as if the breath is coming in through one hand and out through the other. This can be done over the entire body wherever there is tension or pain.

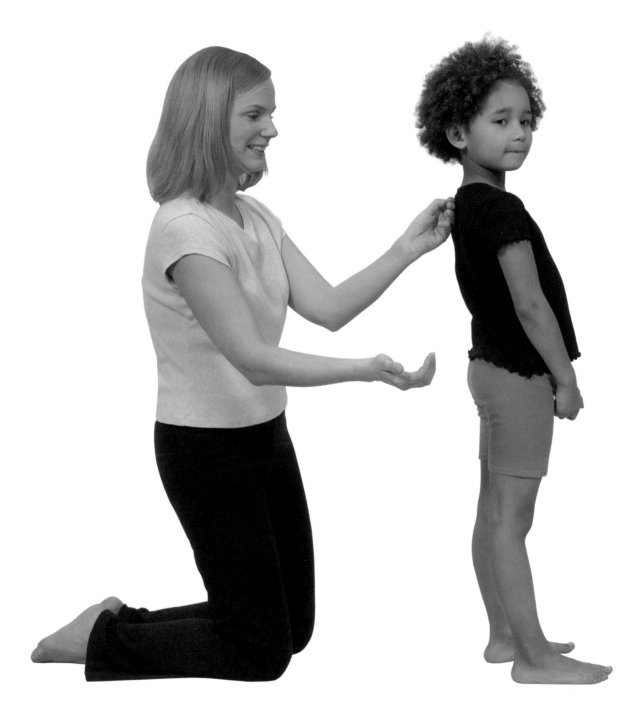

5. kahi la'au the symbol—flowers, leaves, roots
Brush the body from head to foot, imagining that you are using flowers or aromatic leaves.
For extra energy, raise one hand as if it is the leaf of a tree receiving sunlight, place the other
on the body, and transfer energy from the upper to the lower hand using your breath and
imagination.

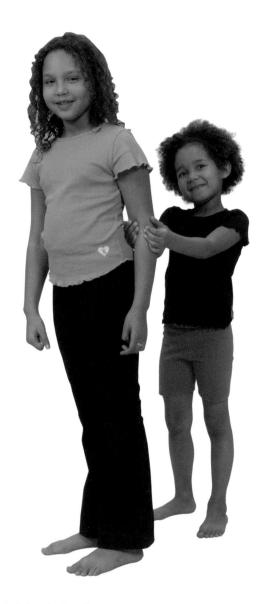

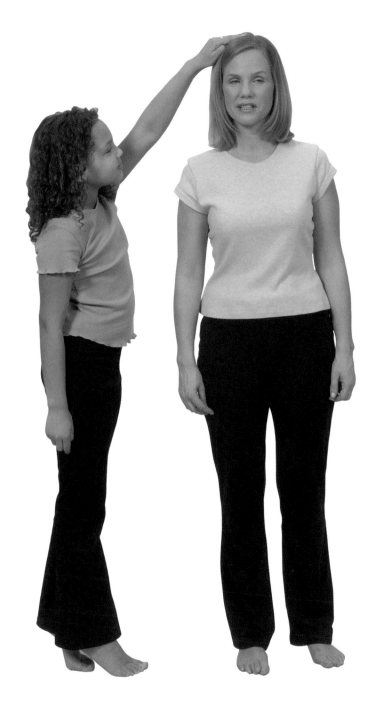

6. kahi holoholona a relaxed animal
Ask your partner to tell you his or her favorite animal and
gently squeeze the body from head to foot in the nature of
that animal. If you can, roll the skin of the back and legs
between your fingers before gently squeezing again.

7. kahi kanaka a loving touch
For one full second on the front only, gently but firmly touch
the crown, brow, throat, solar plexus, and navel. Then using
both hands at once, touch the jaws, elbows, wrists, hips,
knees, ankles, and toes. Finish with a downward sweep
over the invisible aura surrounding the body.

massage for sick and elderly people

As well as bringing with it pain, tension, and often insomnia, illness, particularly when serious in nature, causes worry not just for the patient, but for family and friends too. At such times, close ones have to find ways to cope with their own emotions about the sufferer's state of health, and communication can become strained as people put on a brave face. Being ill can therefore be an isolating experience. A simple massage releases endorphins, the body's natural painkiller, and promotes a form of relaxation that adds to the quality of life of a sick person. It also offers family and friends a very real way to connect. Increasingly, massage is being used in hospices for these very reasons.

massage for older people

Physical touch is a basic human need that elderly people may be lacking, particularly if a partner has died. Even the simplest massage is a concrete expression of care, love, and acceptance.

how to massage

The type of massage you give depends on the nature of the illness or the state of health and physical strength of an elderly person. The seated hand massage shown here develops trust, communication, and eye contact, and may be all that is needed. The seated back massage on page 172, performed clothed and without oil, could be suitable, or try the simple face and foot massage from Part 3. Before you plan the massage, discuss with your partner what he or she would like to receive and what he or she feels comfortable with. Remember that it is the quality of touch and the care and thought behind the touch that is particularly important at this time.

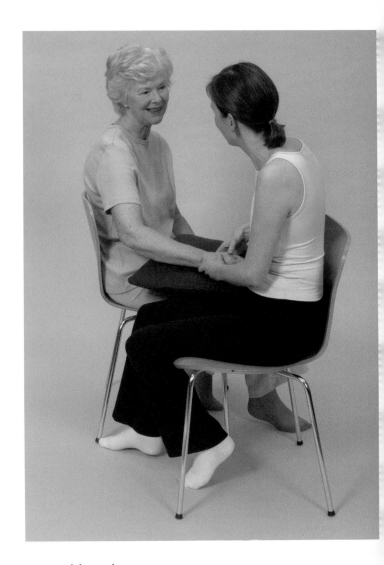

seated hand massage

❶ Sit with your partner's arm resting on a pillow or table, in your lap, or on the side of the bed.

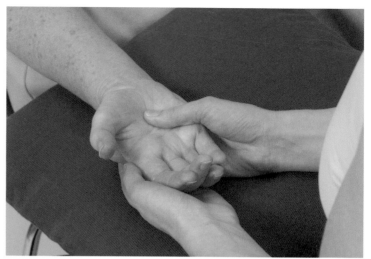

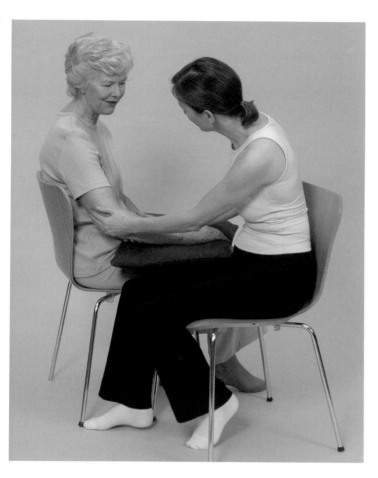

❷ Start by making flowing effleurage strokes over the back of the hand and arm, as demonstrated on page 96.

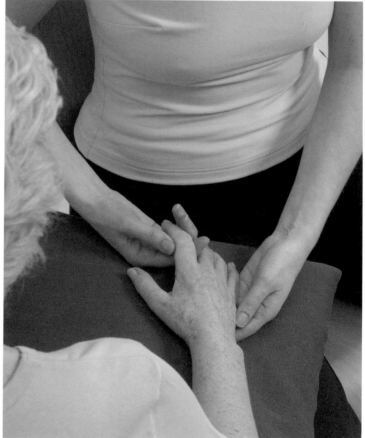

❸ Work around the fingers, as shown on page 97.

❹ Loosen the joints, as shown on page 98.

seated clothed massage

Lying on the front of the body doesn't suit everyone. It may be especially uncomfortable—or downright impossible—for pregnant women, elderly people, and those with back problems. As an alternative, provide a massage with your partner seated on a stool. Most of the techniques from other sections, with the recipient shown in a lying position, can be performed in a sitting position.

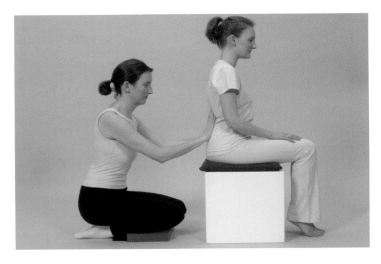

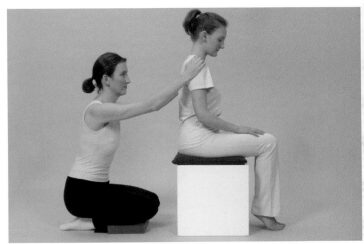

effleurage for the back

❶ Stand or kneel behind your partner. If you're standing, have one foot in front of the other. Place both your hands, fingers and thumbs together and fingers pointing upward, at the base of the lower back on either side of the spine.

❷ Glide your hands up the length of the back, over the top of the shoulders, and down the sides of the back, returning to the starting position to repeat the stroke. Lean in with some body weight to make the stroke firmer, asking your partner for feedback.

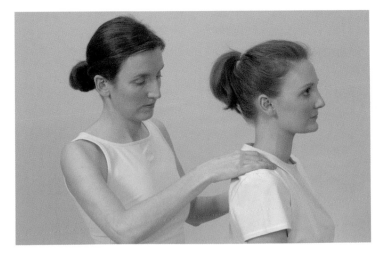

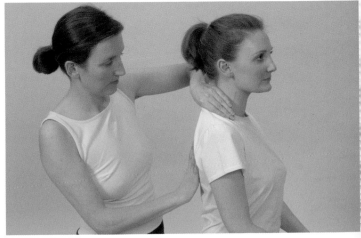

alternate kneading on the upper back

❶ Standing with one foot in front of the other, follow the instructions on page 65. If your partner is clothed, make sure to work over the fabric at all times to prevent friction burns.

❷ Lean forward as you push the muscles away from the bones and transfer your weight to the back foot as you pull back on the muscles. Ask your partner to lift the head slightly to help loosen the shoulder muscles.

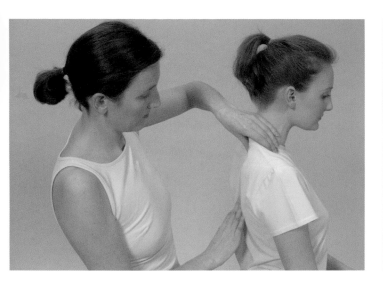

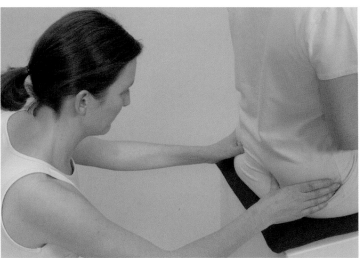

muscle shaking

Remaining in the same standing position, grab the muscle on the top of the shoulder between the fingers and thumb of one or both hands. One or both hands may be used. Repeat on the other shoulder.

spiraling pressure

❶ Kneeling on the floor, on both knees if possible, place your thumbs on either side of the lower back on the gluteal muscles.

❷ Follow the instructions on page 69, leaning in with your body weight on the initial part of the stroke and rocking forward from the knees.

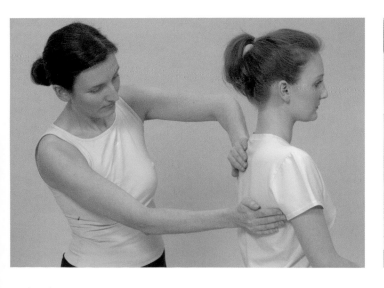

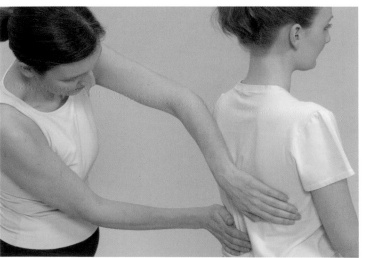

wringing

❶ Standing to the side of your partner, place the flat of each hand, fingers and thumbs together, on each side of the back, starting at the top of the shoulders. Ensure both hands point in the same direction, away from you.

❷ Follow the instructions on page 48, bending slightly to crisscross the hands down and up the length of the back. If this strains your back, omit this technique.

massage for emotional release

It is impossible to touch people physically without touching them emotionally. If you think about how the body tenses up against the forces of a harsh wind, you can begin to understand how it might be possible to have a physical response to harsh words and difficult situations. Some research shows that we have a cellular memory, holding memories of experiences within the body's tissues. Work on these tissues might cause the recipient to experience an opening up, a greater desire to talk about grief or to express difficult or unhappy feelings. Massage is extremely beneficial and supportive during times of emotional upset, grief, and bereavement. It helps the recipient feel cared for and nurtured and offers a safe haven in which to release emotion.

using essential oils

Aromatherapy draws on the medicinal properties of plants, using essential oils derived from a plant to treat physical and emotional ailments or to relax, revitalize, and rebalance. The following oils assist in emotional release and grief: lavender, neroli, bergamot, basil, rosemary, rose, and geranium. Place a few drops on a tissue for your partner to inhale as he or she receives the massage.

how to massage

In times of grief, we need to be treated gently, and this is true also when giving massage. All the massage sequences in Parts 2 and 3 are appropriate for use in times of emotional upset. Place much more emphasis as you work through a massage on stroking techniques, such as effleurage, circling, forearm stroking, feathering, and combing, and on the gentle application of cat paws, wringing, and raking.

If someone cries when you are giving a massage, give reassurance and discontinue the massage for a while, but stay in contact with your partner, offer tissues and a sympathetic ear, and allow the emotional release to happen. Only continue the massage when your partner indicates that he or she is ready to start again.

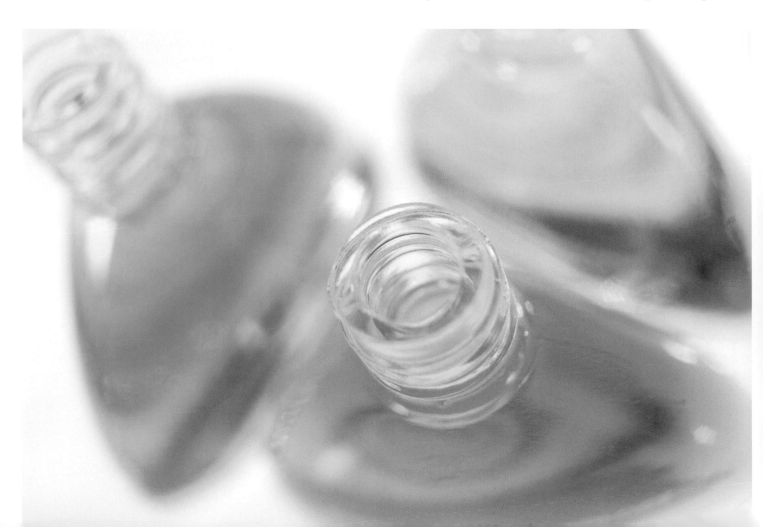

massage at work

There is a growing trend within the workplace for health-related benefits to be supplied as part of a remuneration deal: perhaps membership at a gym, private health insurance, or a corporate medical team. Exercise classes may be held before work, yoga conducted in the boardroom, and on-site massage—a seated, clothed, acupressure technique—given at workers' desks. I run stress-management training for the corporate world; in sessions, we often get up from where we are sitting and incorporate a few fun massage techniques over clothes, standing in a circle. Massage is a great way to break down barriers within an organization and to develop trust. You might like to try the acupressure massage shown here, referring to the map of pressure points as you work. You could also try the seated clothed massage on page 172 and the family massage on page 166.

acupressure massage

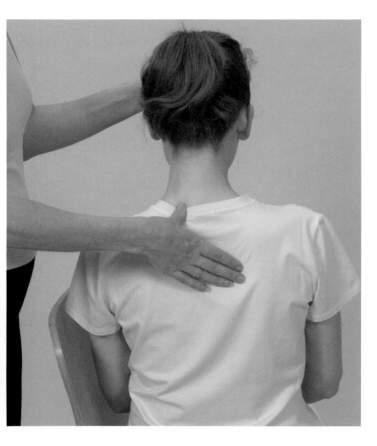

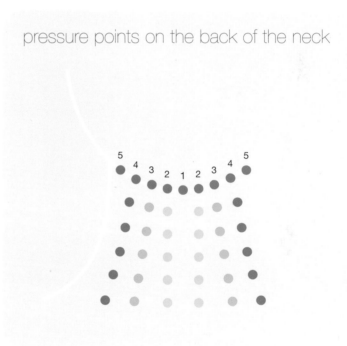

pressure points on the back of the neck

❶ Begin with your partner seated. Stand on his or her left side by the shoulder, facing across the head and shoulders. Use your left hand gently to support the forehead while you massage with your right hand.

❷ Starting at the small indentation at the top of the spine (point 1), apply gentle pressure with your thumb to each point just below the base of the skull (blue dots). Work out from point 1 toward point 5. Repeat this line.

❸ Placing your thumb just below the second point on the skull, gently apply pressure into the muscle, resting your fingers on the opposite side of the neck for support. Work down the neck toward the shoulders, applying pressure to each point (yellow dots). Repeat.

❹ Use the same technique to work down the line, starting just below point 3 (green dots). Work down this line twice.

❺ Repeat, beginning just below point 4 (pink dots). Move around to the other side of your partner and repeat the sequence.

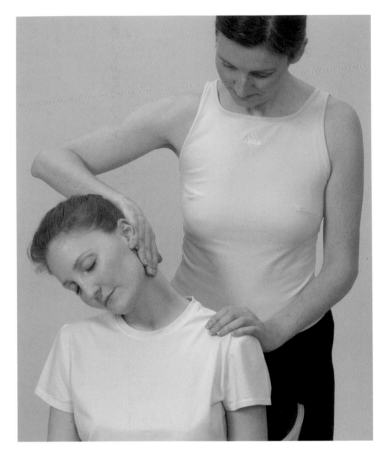

neck stretch

❶ Standing behind your partner, place your left hand on his or her left shoulder. Place your right palm on the left side of the head, just below the ear. Make sure your fingers point down, your elbow straight up.

❷ Gently pull the head over toward the right shoulder until your partner feels an easy stretch. Slowly return the head to center and repeat the stretch to the opposite side.

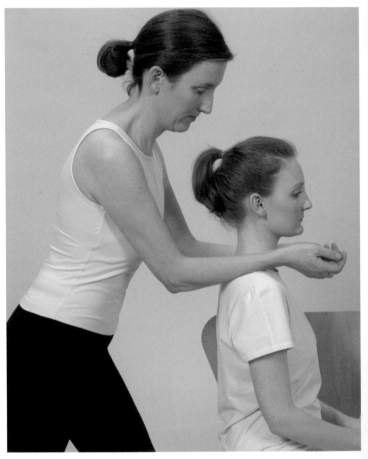

shoulder press

❶ Use your forearms to press down on the top of the shoulders. Start with your arms close to the neck and lean in and down with your body weight.

❷ Move your arms slightly away from the neck and lean in again. Now move out slightly further and lean in once more. Work toward the outer edge of the shoulders.

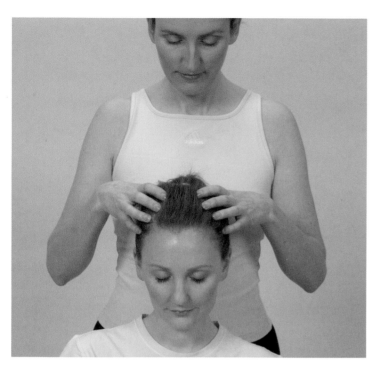

shampooing
❶ Still standing behind your partner, place your fingers on the scalp and gently move them in a circular movement so that the skin moves slightly.

❷ Repeat all over the scalp—imagine you are shampooing the hair.

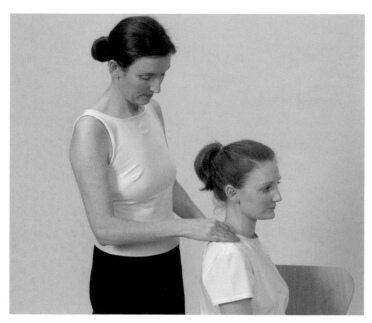

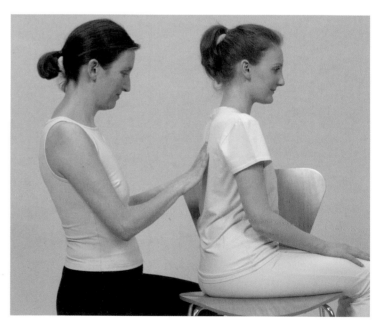

shoulder squeeze
❶ Squeeze your partner's shoulders between your fingers and thumbs. Start close to the neck and work across the shoulders toward the top of the arms.

❷ Squeeze three times down the tops of the arms. Repeat two or three times.

brushing down
❶ With one hand on either side of the spine, use the tips of your fingers to brush down your partner's back from the base of the skull to the lower back in one smooth stroke. Repeat.

❷ Now brush down from the sides of the neck, down the arms to the wrists, and repeat.

massage for jet lag

Cabin pressure, lack of humidity, change of time zone, lack of sleep, alcohol, and dehydration are contributing factors to jet lag. Spend a little time preparing for a flight to minimize the effects. A few days before you fly, avoid alcohol or caffeine and drink plenty of water to ensure the body is well hydrated. Pack in your bag a horseshoe neck pillow, an eye mask and ear plugs, and some socks, and wear several layers of natural-fiber clothing. Self-massage while traveling is a wonderful tool for preventing stiff muscles and ensuring the body remains in good health.

self-help dos and don'ts

- As soon as you board the flight, set your watch to the time of your destination and, as much as possible, eat and sleep according to those times. Eat very lightly.
- Take off your shoes and relax with some deep breathing (page 183). Make yourself as comfortable as possible: the pillow supplied by the airline is useful to give more support to the lower back.
- Avoid alcohol, tea, coffee, and caffeinated soft drinks: they dehydrate the body. Avoid also sleeping pills, which bring about a type of sleep in which you do not move much, increasing the chance of thrombosis. Do not take melatonin; it has adverse side effects.
- Drink plenty of water and use a spray bottle to regularly spritz your face and improve humidity.
- Move around the cabin as often as possible, and while seated, exercise by flexing and extending the feet, circling the ankles, flexing and extending at the knee and hip, rotating the wrists, and circling the neck.
- Massage the buttocks by rolling from side to side in your seat to prevent numbness.
- Studies prove that circadian rhythms can be shifted by exposing the eyes to bright daylight without sunglasses for fifteen minutes.

essential oils for the traveler

Lavender and geranium encourage sleep on a flight, while rosemary and peppermint stimulate on arrival. Place a few drops on a tissue and inhale.

If you suffer from swollen ankles and feet, mix a ratio of 1 drop of peppermint oil to ¾ ounce vegetable oil and massage the legs, as on page 142. Refrain from using this oil if, for example, you are pregnant or taking homeopathic remedies.

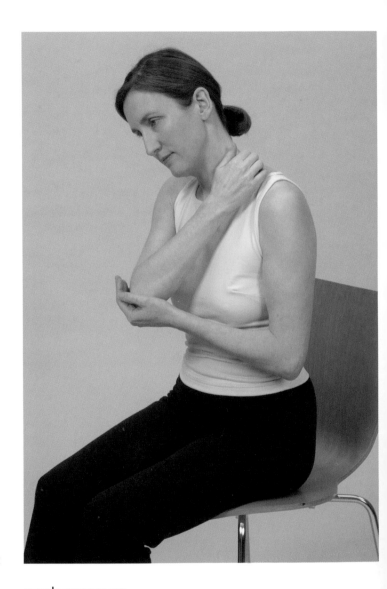

neck pressure
Supporting your arm at the elbow, apply deep, circular strokes into the neck and shoulder on the opposite side with your fingertips.

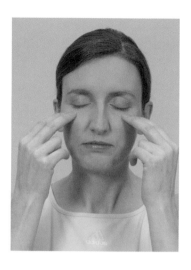
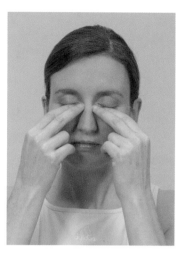
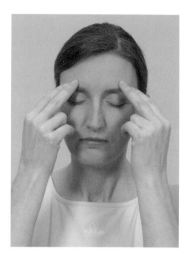
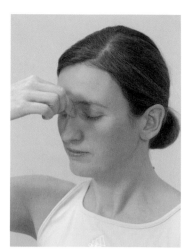

face massage

Make sure you regularly moisturize your face during the flight. Massage moisturizer in by circling around the eyes with gentle fingertip strokes, taking care not to drag the skin. Circle around the cheeks and forehead, then briskly pinch the bridge of the nose to stimulate circulation to the eyes.

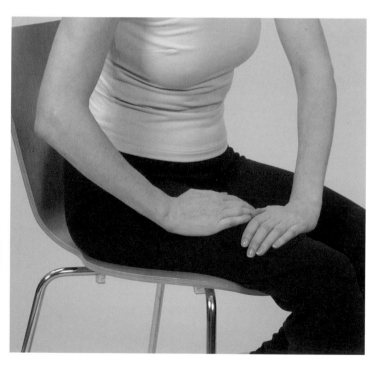

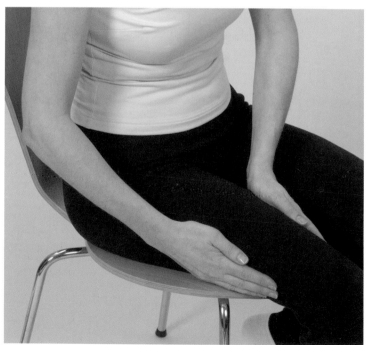

antiswelling massage

❶ Use effleurage (page 142) on the thigh over your clothing, placing emphasis on the upward stroke to encourage fluid that pools in the ankles and causes swelling to circulate around the body.

❷ With both hands, stroke up the thigh from knee to hip, using brisk, sweeping strokes to drain the area.

❸ Repeat on the calf, and then again on the thigh. Repeat all the strokes on the other leg.

massage for cellulite

Cellulite is a contentious issue: there are heated debates over what it is, the causes, and indeed whether it exists. Many complementary therapists subscribe to the theory that the body forms cellulite as a way of dealing with toxins that it cannot eliminate ordinarily because of poor circulation, lack of exercise, and toxic overload. Given that cellulite seems to be a modern-day problem and that quantities of additives and chemicals in our diet now were not common fifty years ago, this theory seems plausible. Massage on its own will not rid the body of cellulite, but combine it with exercise, a good detox followed by a healthy and natural diet, drinking lots of water, and skin brushing to stimulate the lymphatic system, and you should soon see good results.

how it develops

Toxins react with fat cells in the body, causing them to harden, giving the dimpled and lumpy effect around women's thighs and buttocks. Men are more prone to storing this fat around the abdomen.

how to massage

A stimulating massage, encouraging a fresh supply of blood to the area and encouraging the flow of fluids through the body, will help start the breakdown process. Perform all the techniques detailed here much more briskly than normal. Try also the following techniques from Part 2: raking up the thigh, pressure techniques up the thigh, pummeling, cupping, raindrops, and friction rubbing. The self-massage techniques on the leg from Part 4 are also beneficial.

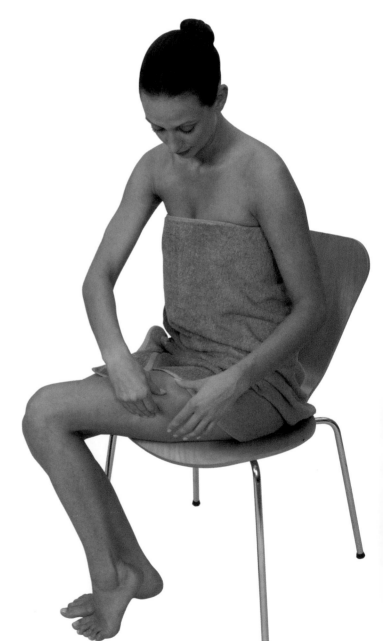

plucking

Pluck the fleshy area of the thigh and buttocks with the fingers and thumbs of both hands alternately, as if plucking the feathers from a chicken.

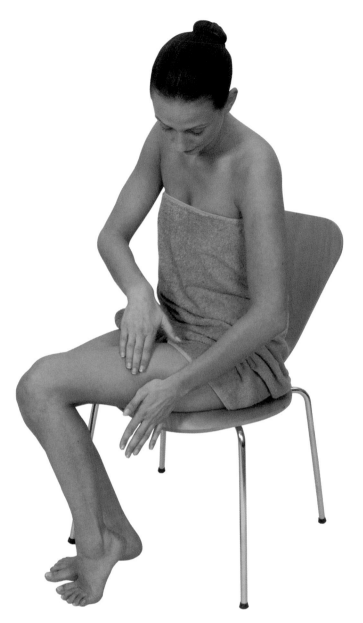

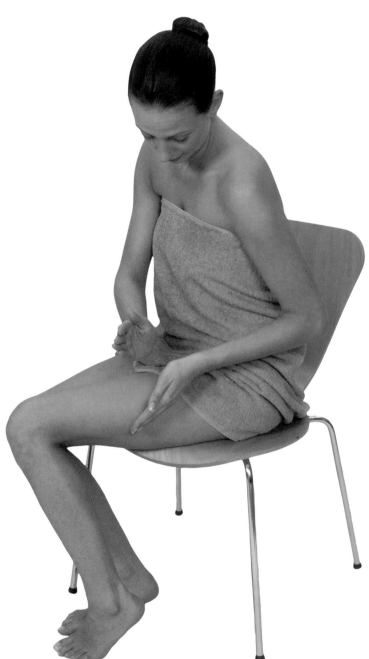

pulling and pushing

❶ With one hand and then the other, pull the fleshy area of the thigh toward you.

❷ Using the heel of the hand, push the flesh back away from you. Repeat the brisk pulling and pushing motion.

hacking

With loose wrists and a firm hand, strike the fleshy area with the blade of each hand alternately. The hands should move so quickly they become a blur.

massage for stress relief

All the techniques in the book are antidotes to stress—massage is one of the best ways of reversing the stress cycle. Whether you receive a massage, give a massage, do some self-massage, or follow the self-help stretching exercises, you will surely feel like a different person afterward. At different times during the day, turn your attention to your breath, using the exercises here to deepen your breathing, slow you down, and reverse the stress cycle.

relaxing essential oils

For help during times of stress, choose lavender, clary sage, neroli, and rose. Place a few drops on a tissue and inhale.

visualization and pressure-point exercise

❶ Remember something you find relaxing, a memory of a vacation, for example. See it, hear any sounds associated with it, smell any fragrances, and remember that feeling of relaxation.

❷ Press with one thumb into the center of your other palm. Find the most sensitive spot and press, even if it is painful. This is an acupressure point for stress relief.

❸ Continue to visualize whatever makes you feel relaxed as you release the pressure.

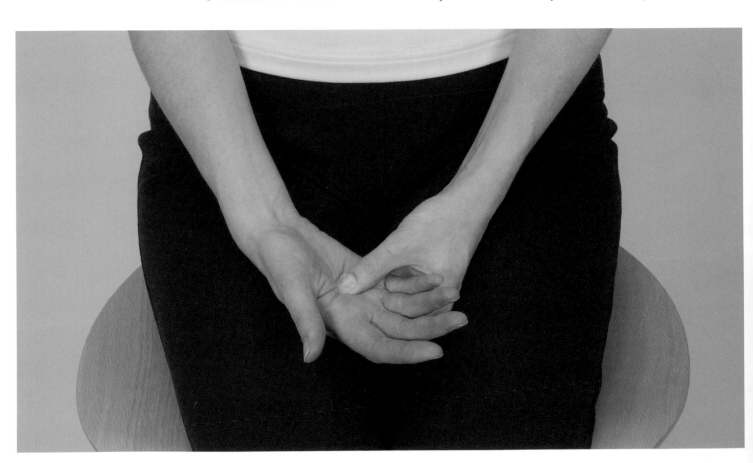

deep breathing exercise

❶ Make sure you are comfortable and relaxed, either sitting in a chair or lying on the floor. Let the chair or floor fully support your weight; sink into it and do not feel that you have to hold yourself up in any way. If sitting in a chair, make sure you avoid slumping.

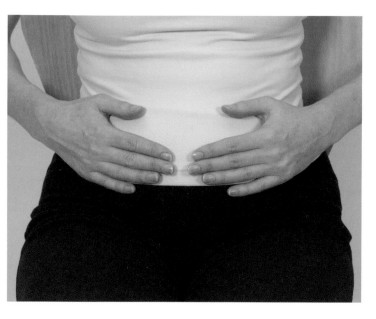 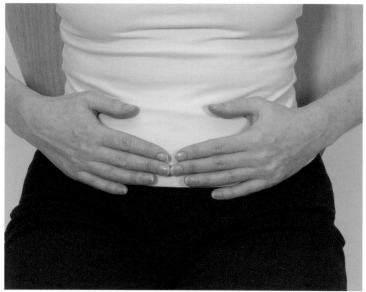

❷ Allow your shoulders to relax and place your hands over your abdomen so your fingertips touch slightly. Take a nice, deep breath in. As you breathe in, notice how the fingertips of each hand separate. Your abdomen is expanding, indicating that you are breathing fully, using the diaphragm muscle beneath the ribs to initiate the breath.

❸ As you breathe out, feel your abdomen relax and your fingertips come together again.

❹ Repeat, counting slowly to four as you breathe in and again as you breathe out. Gradually slow the counting so that your breaths become slower and deeper.

❺ Once you feel comfortable with the technique, try holding for a few seconds between the breath in and the breath out.

anatomy

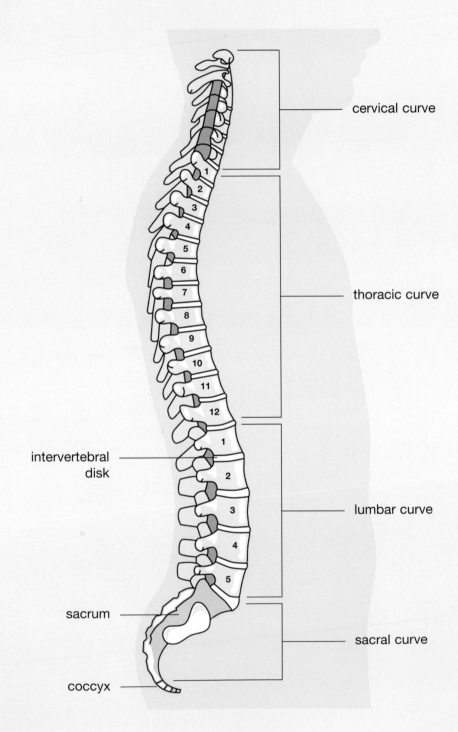

the spine

cervical curve

thoracic curve

intervertebral disk

lumbar curve

sacrum

sacral curve

coccyx

the digestive system

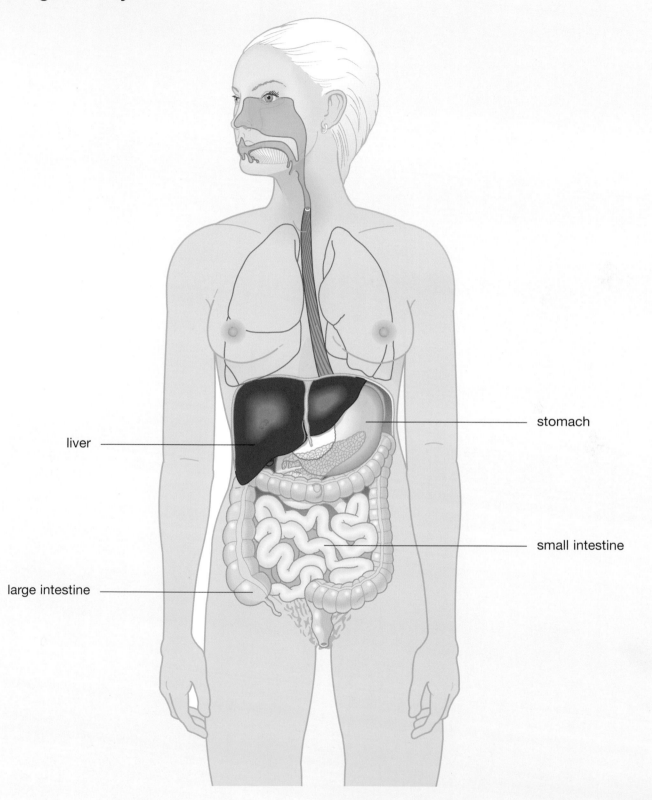

liver

stomach

small intestine

large intestine

main muscle groups (front)

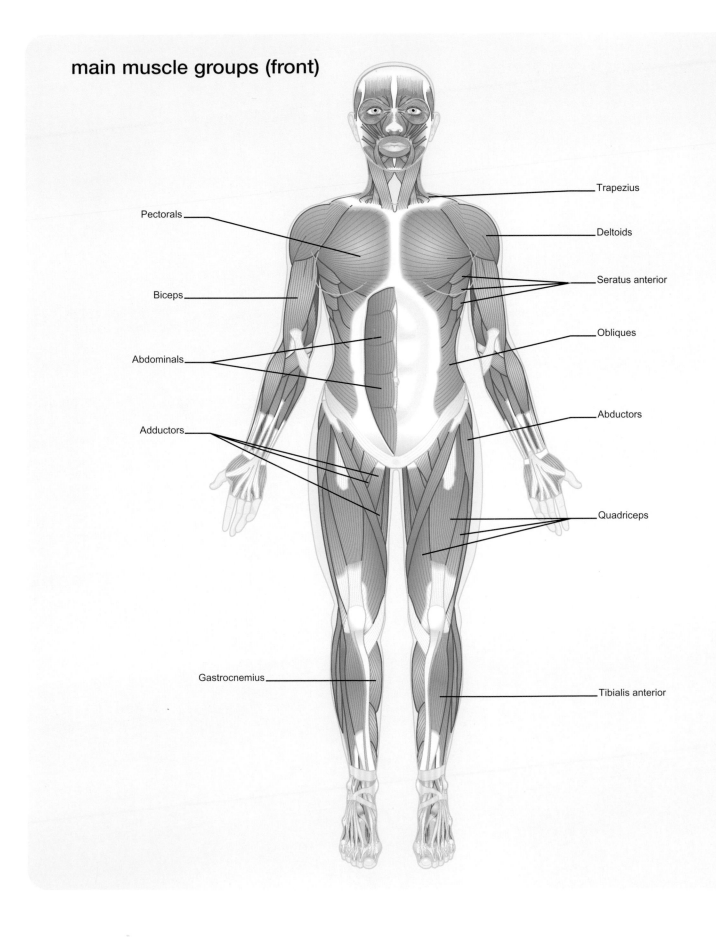

Trapezius

Pectorals

Deltoids

Seratus anterior

Biceps

Obliques

Abdominals

Abductors

Adductors

Quadriceps

Gastrocnemius

Tibialis anterior

main muscle groups (back)

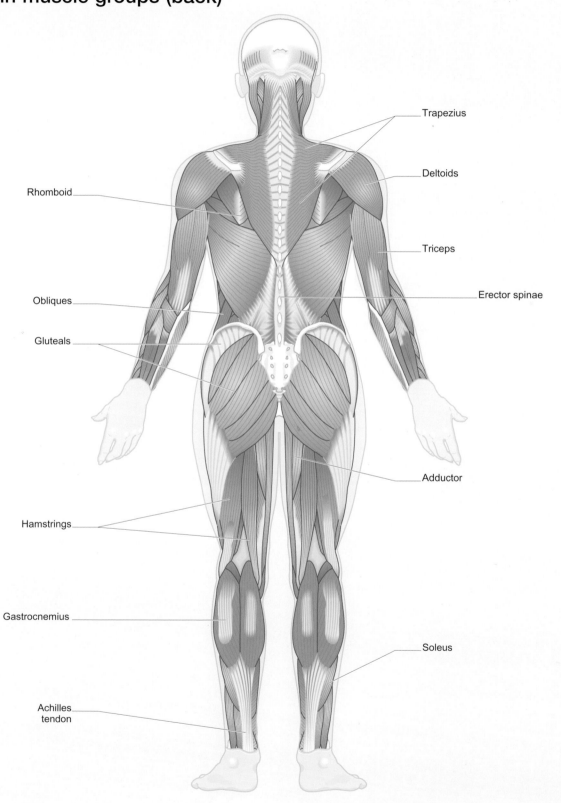

Trapezius

Deltoids

Rhomboid

Triceps

Obliques

Erector spinae

Gluteals

Adductor

Hamstrings

Gastrocnemius

Soleus

Achilles tendon

resources

United States

massage organizations

American Massage Therapy Association
820 Davis Street, Suite 100
Evanston, IL 60201-4444
Tel: 847-864-0123

International Massage Association
P.O. Drawer 421
Warrenton, VA 20188-0421
Tel: 540-351-0800
www.imagroup.com
e-mail: info@imagroup.com

Associated Bodyworker and Massage Professionals
1271 Sugarbush Drive
Evergreen, CO 80439-9766
Tel: 800-458-2267
www.abmp.com
e-mail: expectmore@abmp.com

American Holistic Health Association
P.O. Box 17400
Anaheim, CA 92817-7400
Tel: 714-779-6152
www.ahha.org
e-mail: ahha@healthy.net

American Medical Massage Association
P.O. Box 272
Gainesville, VA 20156-0272
Tel: 540-351-0807
Fax: 540-351-0041
www.americanmedicalmassage.com
e-mail: rdeperio@americanmedicalmassage.com

Association of Massage Therapists–New South Wales
25 South East Kings Bay Drive
Crystal River, FL 34429
Tel: 352-795-2081

International Aromatherapy and Herb Association
3541 West Acapulco Lane
Phoenix, AZ 85053
Tel: 602-938-4439

International Association for Holistic Aromatherapy
2000 Second Avenue, #206
Seattle, WA 98121
Tel: 888-ASK-NAHA
www.naha.org
e-mail: info@naha.org

International Thai Therapists Association
47 West Polk Street, #100-329
Chicago, IL 60605
Tel: 773-792-4121
www.thaimassage.com
e-mail: itta@megsinet.net

National AIDS Massage Project
215 West 24th Street
Minneapolis, MN 55404-3202
Tel: 612-874-9768

National Board of Reflexology
2380 Bellbrook Avenue
Xenia, OH 45385
Tel: 937-708-3232

Nursing Touch & Massage Therapy Association International
737 Robert Boulevard, Suite 1
Slidell, LA 70458
Tel: 540-893-8002

Reflexology Association of America
4012 South Rainbow Boulevard
P. O. Box K585
Las Vegas, NV 89103-2059
Tel: 702-871-9522
www.reflexology-USA.org

Reiki Alliance
P.O. Box 41
Cataldo, ID 83810
Tel: 208-783-3535

baby massage

International Association of Infant Massage
1891 Goodyear Avenue, Suite #622
Ventura, CA 93003
Tel: 800-248-5432
Fax: 805-644-7699
www.iaim-us.com
e-mail: iaim4us@aol.com

National Association of Pregnancy Massage Therapy
1007 Mopoc Circle
Austin, TX 78758
Tel: 888-451-4945

elderly massage

Service Through Touch–Skilled
Touch for the Elderly, Ill and Dying
41 Carl Street, Suite C
San Francisco, CA 94117
Tel: 415-564-1750
www.sf-care.n3.net

magazines

Massage Magazine
www.massagemag.com

Inbalance Magazine
www.inbalancemagazine.com

Massage World
Subscribe via www.amazon.com

books

Care Through Massage
Mary Ann Finch
The Continuum Publishing Company

Infant Massage: A Handbook for Loving Parents
Vimala McClure
Bantam Books

Aromatherapy Massage: Harnessing the Powers of Essential Oils and Therapeutic Touch Techniques
Sarah Porter
Southwater Publications

The Book of Massage: The Complete Step-by-Step Guide to Eastern and Western Techniques
Lucy Lidell, Lucinda Lidell, Sara Thomas, Carola Beresford-Cooke
Fireside

The Complete Book of Massage
Clare Maxwell-Hudson
Random House

United Kingdom

massage schools

Essentials for Health
11–15 High Street
Marlow
Bucks SL17 1AU
Tel: 0845 108 0088
www.essentialsforhealth.co.uk
e-mail: enquiries@essentialsforhealth.co.uk

Institute of Complementary Medicine
P.O. Box 194
London SE16 1QZ
Tel: 020 7237 5165

British Complementary Medicine Association
P.O. Box 5122
Bournemouth BH8 0WG
Tel: 0845 345 5977
e-mail: info@bcma.co.uk

Complementary Medical Association
67 Eagle Heights
The Falcons
Bramlands Close
London SW11 2LJ
Tel: 0845 129 8434
www.the-cma.org.uk

Association of Holistic Biodynamic Massage Therapists

42 Catharine Street

Cambridge CB1 3AW

Tel: 01223 240 815

www.ahbmt.co.uk

e-mail: kathrin@ahbmt.co.uk

General Council for Massage Therapy

46 Millhead Way

Hertford

Hertfordshire SG14 3YH

Tel: 01992 537637

www.gcmt-uk.org

Massage Therapy Institute of Great Britain

PO Box 2726

London NW2 3NR

Tel: 0208 2081607

www.cmhmassage.co.uk/mtigb.htm

Complementary Health Information Service

www.chisuk.org.uk

on-site massage

Hands on People

Tel: 020 7352 5262

Fax: 020 7352 5033

www.handsonpeople.co.uk

e-mail: info@handsonpeople.co.uk

The Academy of On-Site Massage

Avon Road

Charfield

Wotton-under-Edge

Gloucestershire GL12 8TT

Tel: 01454 261900

www.aosm.co.uk

lomi lomi

Stenhouse Consultancy

36 Plasturton Gdns

Pontcanna

Cardiff CF11 9HF

Tel: 02920 377723.

www.hawaiianlomilomi.co.uk

e-mail: realatsten@aol.com

baby massage and massage in pregnancy

International Association of Infant Massage

56 Sparsholt Road

Barking

Essex IG11 7YQ

Tel: 0208 5911399

www.iaim.org.uk

e-mail: mail@iaim.org.uk

acknowledgments

Pregnancy massage text reproduced by kind permission of Suzanne Yates of Wellmother.
Lomi lomi massage reproduced by kind permission of Liz Newton of the Stenhouse Consultancy.
Seated massage techniques reproduced by kind permission of Alisdair Burcher of Touch Pro.

index

References in *italics* indicate specific
massage techniques